Beating Restless Legs Syndrome Naturally

Scott A. Johnson

Beating Restless Legs Syndrome Naturally / Scott A. Johnson

Cover design: Scott A. Johnson

ISBN-13: 978-1-972974-04-9

Published by Scott A. Johnson Professional Writing Services, LLC: Orem, UT

Discover more books by Scott A. Johnson at authorscott.com/shop/

DISCLAIMERS OF WARRANTY AND LIMITATION OF LIABILITY

The author provides all information on an "as is" and "as available" basis and for informational purposes only. The author makes no representations or warranties of any kind, expressed or implied, as to the information, materials, or products mentioned. Every effort has been made to ensure accuracy and completeness of the information contained; however, it is not intended to replace any medical advice or to halt proper medical treatment, nor diagnose, treat, cure, or prevent any health condition or disease. Always consult a qualified medical professional before using any dietary supplement or natural product, engaging in physical activity, or modifying your diet; and seek the advice of your physician with any questions you may have regarding any medical condition.

Always consult your OB/GYN if you are pregnant or think you may become pregnant before using any dietary supplement or natural product, and to ensure you are healthy enough for exercise or any dietary modifications. The information contained in this book is for educational and informational purposes only, and it is not meant to replace medical advice, diagnosis, or treatment in any manner. Never delay or disregard professional medical advice. Use the information solely at your own risk; the author accepts no responsibility for the use thereof. This book is sold with the understanding that neither the author nor publisher shall be liable for any loss, injury, or harm allegedly arising from any information or suggestion in this book.

The Food and Drug Administration (FDA) has not evaluated the statements contained in this book. The information and materials are not meant to diagnose, prescribe, or treat any disease, condition, illness, or injury. You are encouraged to seek the most current information and medical care from your healthcare professional.

CONTENTS

CHAPTER ONE

WHAT IS RLS—REALLY?

You lie down after a long day, ready for sleep. But within minutes, something starts happening in your legs. It's hard to describe—not quite pain, not quite an itch, more like a deep, restless crawling sensation that will not stop. The only thing that helps is getting up and moving. So you do. And for a moment, it goes away. But the second you lie back down, it starts again.

If that sounds familiar, you are not imagining things. You are not being dramatic. And you are definitely not alone. What you are experiencing has a name: Restless Legs Syndrome, or RLS—and it affects hundreds of millions of people worldwide.[1]

And yet, for a condition that common, RLS remains one of the most misunderstood, misdiagnosed, and underappreciated conditions in modern medicine. In this chapter, we will cut through the confusion and give you a clear, honest picture of what RLS actually is—starting from the ground up.

The Official Definition—and Why It Falls Short

Medically speaking, RLS is classified as a neurological sensory-movement disorder. The key phrase there is sensory-movement—

meaning it affects both how you feel (sensations in your legs) and how your body responds to those feelings (an overwhelming urge to move).

The official diagnostic criteria, set by the International Restless Legs Syndrome Study Group, include four core features:

- An urge to move the legs, usually accompanied by uncomfortable sensations
- Symptoms that start or get worse during rest or inactivity
- Symptoms that are partially or totally relieved by movement
- Symptoms that are worse in the evening or at night

That is the textbook version. But if you have lived with RLS, you know the definition barely scratches the surface of what it actually feels like—or what it actually costs you.

What RLS Actually Feels Like

One of the reasons RLS is so frequently dismissed—by doctors, by family members, even by the people who have it—is that the sensations are genuinely difficult to describe. They do not fit neatly into words like "pain" or "cramp." Most people cycle through several descriptions before landing on one that feels even close:

- A crawling or creeping sensation under the skin
- Tingling, like electricity moving through the limb
- A deep itch that cannot be scratched
- Tension or tightness that demands release
- A pulling or tugging sensation inside the legs
- A feeling of restlessness that seems to come from the bones themselves

While the legs are most commonly affected, some people also experience these sensations in the arms, torso, or even the face, though this is less common. The important distinction from muscle cramps or nerve pain is that movement—walking, stretching, rubbing the legs—actually helps, at least temporarily. That defining feature of temporary relief with movement is one of the clearest clinical signals that what someone is experiencing is RLS and not something else.

> *The urge to move is not just uncomfortable—it is compulsive. Many people describe it as feeling impossible to resist, almost like holding your breath. You can fight it for a little while, but eventually, you simply have to move.*

Why Nighttime Is the Worst

There is a reason RLS is primarily a sleep disorder as much as a movement disorder. Symptoms are consistently and significantly worse in the evening and at night—typically peaking between 10 p.m. and 4 a.m. This is not coincidence, and it is not just because you happen to notice it more when you are trying to sleep.

There are real biological reasons for this circadian pattern. The brain chemical dopamine—which plays a central role in RLS, as we will explore in depth in the next chapter—naturally dips in the evening. Body temperature also drops as part of the natural wind-down toward sleep, which may affect nerve signaling. And the iron that your brain depends on to regulate movement control fluctuates throughout the day, reaching its lowest point in the late evening.

Put those factors together, and the biological deck is stacked against RLS sufferers every evening. The result is a cruel paradox: The time when you most need to be still and rest is the exact time your legs seem most intent on rebellion.

The Real Cost: Sleep Deprivation and Beyond

To understand why RLS matters—really matters—you have to look past the legs and consider what chronic sleep disruption does to a person over time.

Most people with moderate to severe RLS struggle to fall asleep, wake repeatedly throughout the night, or experience what researchers call sleep fragmentation—where the brain keeps getting pulled out of deep, restorative sleep to process the sensations in the legs. The sleep you do get is simply not as good.

The downstream effects of that chronic sleep deprivation are significant and wide-ranging:

- **Fatigue and low energy** that does not improve with rest
- **Brain fog** and difficulty concentrating
- **Mood changes**—irritability, anxiety, and low mood are common companions of RLS
- **Impaired immune function** from insufficient deep sleep
- **Increased cardiovascular risk**—research increasingly links chronic RLS with elevated blood pressure and heart health concerns[2]
- **Reduced quality of life**—difficulty traveling, socializing, or even sitting through a movie or a meal without discomfort

That last point is worth dwelling on for a moment. RLS does not just happen at night. For people with moderate to severe symptoms, the anticipation of an evening of disrupted sleep can color the entire day. Long car rides, flights, movies, concerts, dinner parties—anything that requires sitting still for an extended period can become something to dread rather than enjoy. Over time, this shapes how people live, what they do, and even how they see themselves.

This is not a minor inconvenience. RLS, at its worst, is genuinely life-limiting.

How RLS Presents: The Spectrum from Mild to Severe

RLS is not one-size-fits-all. It exists on a spectrum, and where you fall on that spectrum can vary over time and in response to lifestyle, health status, and other factors.

Mild RLS

Symptoms occur occasionally—perhaps a few times per month. They are uncomfortable but manageable, and the person can usually fall asleep after some movement or stretching. Many people in this category do not even realize they have a named condition. They just think they are restless sleepers or that their legs are "weird."

Moderate RLS

Symptoms occur at least a few times per week. Sleep quality is noticeably affected. The person is aware that something is wrong and may have started to adapt their schedule or habits around their symptoms—going to bed later to minimize lying-awake time, for example, or avoiding evening activities that require sitting.

Severe RLS

Symptoms occur nightly or nearly every night, often for hours. Sleep is severely disrupted, and daytime functioning suffers as a result. In severe cases, symptoms may also begin appearing during the day—during long periods of sitting at work, on planes, or in meetings. At this stage, RLS is a significant disability.

Intermittent vs. Chronic RLS

Some people experience RLS in episodes—it flares up for a period, then quiets down, sometimes for months at a time. This is called intermittent RLS, and it often follows patterns tied to life circumstances: illness, stress, hormonal shifts, or nutritional changes. Other people deal with symptoms persistently, week after week, year after year. This chronic pattern tends to worsen gradually over time, particularly if the underlying causes are not addressed.

Understanding which pattern you are dealing with matters, because it gives you important clues about what is driving your symptoms. A sudden onset of RLS, or a dramatic worsening after years of mild symptoms, is often a signal that something specific has changed—a new medication, a dietary shift, pregnancy, or a health event worth investigating.

Associated Conditions: RLS Does Not Occur in Isolation

One of the most important things to understand about RLS is that it rarely appears in a vacuum. It tends to cluster with certain other conditions, and recognizing those connections can be a powerful diagnostic clue—and a meaningful guide to treatment.

Pregnancy

RLS affects roughly one in four pregnant women, with symptoms peaking in the third trimester.[3] The connection is almost certainly tied to iron depletion—the growing baby places enormous demands on maternal iron stores—as well as folate and hormonal changes. The good news is that pregnancy-related RLS often resolves after delivery, though it can persist in women who remain iron-depleted postpartum.

Kidney Disease and Dialysis

People with chronic kidney disease, particularly those on dialysis, have some of the highest rates of RLS of any population—estimates range from 20 to 50 percent.[4] Kidney disease disrupts iron metabolism, creates uremia (a buildup of waste products in the blood), and impairs the body's ability to regulate a host of minerals and neurotransmitters. This population tends to have some of the most severe and treatment-resistant RLS, highlighting just how central metabolic health is to this condition.

Iron Deficiency Anemia

There is a well-established link between iron deficiency anemia and RLS.[5] However—and this is a point we will return to repeatedly in this guide—the relationship between iron and RLS is more nuanced than simply "low iron equals RLS." Many people with RLS have iron levels that fall within the "normal" range on standard lab tests. The problem, as we will explore in depth, is not always how much iron is in the blood, but how much iron is reaching the brain.

Peripheral Neuropathy

Nerve damage in the legs and feet—from diabetes, nutritional deficiencies, or other causes—can overlap with RLS or mimic some of its symptoms.[6] Distinguishing between the two matters, because the root causes and most effective approaches differ.

Mental Health Conditions

Anxiety and depression are both more common among people with RLS, though the relationship is bidirectional—meaning poor sleep from RLS can worsen mental health, and underlying mental health conditions can amplify the nervous system overactivation that drives RLS symptoms.[7] Certain antidepressants, particularly selective serotonin reuptake inhibitors (SSRIs), are also known to worsen RLS,[8] which adds a layer of complexity for people dealing with both conditions.

RLS and Periodic Limb Movement Disorder

It is worth briefly mentioning a related condition that often travels alongside RLS: Periodic Limb Movement Disorder, or PLMD.[9] Where RLS involves uncomfortable sensations that drive voluntary movement, PLMD involves involuntary repetitive limb movements that happen during sleep—usually rhythmic kicks or twitches of the legs, occurring every 20 to 40 seconds. Most people with PLMD have no idea it is happening; their partners usually notice it first.

The majority of people with RLS also have PLMD, and the two conditions appear to share underlying mechanisms.[10,11] Addressing the root causes of RLS typically improves PLMD as well, which is another reason why a whole-body approach to treatment is more effective than targeting any single symptom in isolation.

Why Diagnosis Is So Often Delayed

Despite being relatively common, RLS is frequently missed or misdiagnosed. There are a few reasons for this.

First, there is no diagnostic test for RLS. There is no blood panel, no imaging study, no nerve conduction test that confirms it. Diagnosis is entirely clinical—based on a conversation about symptoms. That means it depends on the person reporting their symptoms accurately, and on the clinician knowing what to listen for.

Second, people often minimize or dismiss their own symptoms. Many who have lived with mild to moderate RLS for years have simply adapted to it. They assume it is just how they are built, or they chalk it up to stress or aging. By the time they mention it to a doctor, they may describe it so casually that it does not register as a significant complaint.

Third, RLS symptoms can look like other things. Growing pains in children. Anxiety in adults. Fibromyalgia. Circulatory problems. Neuropathy. Without a thorough understanding of the specific sensory-movement pattern of RLS, it is easy to mistake it for something else—or to attribute the sleep disruption to something unrelated.

If you have been told your symptoms are "just stress," or that "everyone's legs feel that way sometimes," or that you should "just try to relax"—know that your experience is real, it has a name, and there are real, evidence-based explanations for what is happening in your body.

> *RLS is not a character flaw. It is not anxiety dressed up as a physical symptom. It is not something you have to simply endure. It is a real neurological condition with identifiable biological drivers—and as you will discover throughout this guide, those drivers can be addressed.*

Primary vs. Secondary RLS

Clinicians sometimes divide RLS into two categories: primary (or idiopathic) RLS and secondary RLS.

Primary RLS is the term used when no clear underlying cause can be identified. It tends to run in families—there is a meaningful genetic component—and it often begins earlier in life. If you have a parent or sibling with RLS, your own risk is significantly elevated.

Secondary RLS arises as a consequence of another identifiable condition or factor—iron deficiency, kidney disease, pregnancy, certain medications, or nutritional deficiencies. In these cases, addressing the underlying cause often significantly improves or resolves the RLS.

Here is what is important to understand, though: The distinction between primary and secondary RLS is less clear-cut than it used to seem. Modern research suggests that even so-called "primary" RLS typically involves identifiable biological disruptions—particularly in iron metabolism and dopamine regulation. The label "idiopathic" often means we have not looked hard enough yet, not that there is no cause to find.

This is one of the core principles of this guide: RLS is not random, and it is not inevitable. There are reasons your nervous system is sending these distress signals—and when you understand those reasons, you can do something about them.

What You Need to Take Away from This Chapter

Before we move into the science of why RLS happens, let us anchor a few foundational truths that will inform everything that follows:

- **RLS is real.** It is a recognized neurological condition, not an imagined one.
- **The symptoms are distinct.** The crawling, tingling, restless urge to move—worse at night, relieved by movement—is a specific, identifiable pattern.
- **The impact is real.** Chronic sleep disruption from RLS has measurable consequences for health, mood, and quality of life.
- **RLS has causes.** It is not a random misfire. The next chapter will show you exactly what is happening in the brain when RLS strikes—and why the conventional explanation has always been only part of the story.

You have spent long enough trying to sleep through something that is actively working against your rest. It is time to understand what you are actually dealing with—and then start addressing it at its source.

• • •

In Chapter 2, we go inside the brain to uncover what science now tells us is really driving RLS—and why the old story was always missing a crucial piece.

CHAPTER TWO

THE ROOT CAUSE—UPDATED SCIENCE

For decades, if you walked into a doctor's office and were diagnosed with RLS, you were handed a fairly simple explanation: Your brain is not making enough dopamine, so your legs are restless. The fix, therefore, was to give the brain more dopamine—or at least mimic its effects with medication.

That explanation was not entirely wrong. Dopamine absolutely plays a role in RLS. The problem is that it is only a fraction of the story—and treating it as the whole story is precisely why so many people find that their symptoms eventually get worse on medication, not better.

The science has moved on significantly. What researchers now understand about RLS is more nuanced, more actionable, and far more hopeful than the old dopamine story ever was. This chapter walks you through that updated picture—in plain language, without the clinical jargon.

The Dopamine Story–How It Started

Dopamine is one of the brain's most important chemical messengers. It plays a central role in movement, motivation, reward, and the regulation of sensory signals. In Parkinson's disease—a condition characterized by the progressive loss of dopamine-producing brain cells—movement becomes stiff, slow, and difficult. When scientists noticed that the same class of medications used to treat Parkinson's also relieved RLS symptoms, the obvious conclusion seemed to be that RLS must be a dopamine problem.

And it worked. At least at first. Dopamine-based medications—known as dopaminergic agents—typically bring fast, meaningful relief for people with RLS.[12] For a while, this felt like confirmation that the dopamine theory was correct.

But then something troubling started happening. After months or years on these medications, many people found that their symptoms came back—and not just at the same level. They came back worse. Symptoms that had only appeared at night began creeping into the afternoon. Then the morning. Some people found their arms were now involved. The medication doses had to be increased just to achieve the same relief, and even then, the relief was less complete than it used to be.

This phenomenon has a name: augmentation. It is so well-documented and so common with dopaminergic RLS medications that it is now listed as a major clinical concern. Augmentation is not a side effect in the ordinary sense—it is a fundamental problem with the approach. When you repeatedly flood the brain with dopamine signals without addressing why those signals are dysregulated in the first place, the brain compensates by becoming less sensitive to dopamine over time. The underlying problem is not only left unsolved—it is often made worse.

> *Dopamine medications for RLS work like turning up the volume on a radio to drown out static. For a while, it helps. But it does not fix the static—and eventually, even maximum volume is not enough.*

The Modern Understanding–Iron Is the Root Issue

The pivotal shift in RLS research came when scientists stopped asking "Why is dopamine low?" and started asking "What controls dopamine in the first place?" The answer, it turns out, is iron.

Iron is not just a nutrient your red blood cells need to carry oxygen. It is an essential cofactor in a staggering number of biological processes—including the production and regulation of dopamine in the brain.[13] The enzyme responsible for manufacturing dopamine, called tyrosine hydroxylase, cannot function without iron.[14] Iron is also critical to the receptors that dopamine binds to.[15] Without adequate iron in the right brain regions, the entire dopamine signaling system begins to break down.

Think of it this way: Dopamine is the messenger, but iron is what makes the messaging system function. If the brain is short on iron, the dopamine system becomes unreliable—not because the brain has stopped making dopamine, but because it lacks the fundamental resource needed to regulate it properly.

This understanding has been reinforced by brain imaging studies showing that people with RLS have significantly lower iron concentrations in a region of the brain called the substantia nigra—one of the key hubs of dopamine production and movement regulation.[16] Critically, many of these individuals had blood iron levels that appeared normal on routine lab work. The deficit was not in the blood. It was specifically in the brain.

Brain Iron vs. Blood Iron—A Crucial Distinction

This is one of the most important concepts in this entire guide, so it is worth taking a moment to really understand it.

The brain sits behind what is called the blood-brain barrier—a highly selective filtering system that tightly controls what enters the brain from the bloodstream. Iron does not simply drift into brain tissue the way it circulates through the rest of the body. It has to be actively transported across that barrier using specific carrier proteins.[17] If that transport system is not working efficiently—for reasons we will explore in the next chapter—iron can be relatively adequate in the blood and still be critically low in the brain.

This is why a standard blood test showing "normal" iron or even "normal" ferritin and transferrin can be so misleading for people with RLS. The blood and the brain are not the same compartment. A doctor looking only at a routine iron panel is essentially checking whether there is fuel in the gas tank, without checking whether that fuel is actually reaching the engine.

The specific marker that is most useful for understanding iron status in RLS is ferritin—the protein that stores iron in tissues. Research consistently shows that RLS symptoms tend to be more severe in people with lower ferritin levels, even when those levels are technically within the "normal" reference range. The clinically meaningful threshold for RLS appears to be considerably higher than what most standard labs flag as deficient. This is a gap between reference ranges and optimal ranges—and it matters enormously for anyone trying to understand their own condition.

> *Iron is the key that allows the brain to regulate movement and calm signals. Without enough of it in the right places, the whole system becomes unstable—and no amount of dopamine medication can substitute for the missing key.*

The Iron-Dopamine Chain–How It All Connects

With the iron-brain connection established, the dopamine picture becomes much clearer. Here is the chain of events:

- Brain iron falls below the threshold needed for optimal dopamine production and regulation.
- Dopamine synthesis falters. More critically, dopamine receptors—particularly in the movement-control regions of the brain—become less sensitive and less numerous.
- The brain's ability to send smooth, coordinated "stay calm and still" signals to the legs deteriorates.
- The nervous system becomes overactivated—generating those relentless crawling, tingling sensations and the overwhelming urge to move.

Notice where the breakdown originates: not in the dopamine system itself, but upstream of it, at the level of iron availability. That is why treating dopamine alone—without addressing the iron deficit—is like treating the smoke without putting out the fire.

This chain also helps explain the genetic dimension of RLS. Several of the genes associated with a higher risk of developing RLS are involved in iron metabolism and transport—not in dopamine production directly.[18,19] The genetic predisposition to RLS appears to be, in large part, a predisposition to brain iron insufficiency.

Enter Glutamate—The Brain's Accelerator Pedal

Dopamine and iron are only part of the updated RLS picture. In recent years, researchers have identified another key player: glutamate.[20,21]

Glutamate is the brain's primary excitatory neurotransmitter—meaning it is the chemical that activates and stimulates neurons. If dopamine is the system that helps regulate and coordinate movement, glutamate is what sends the "go" signal. In a well-functioning nervous system, excitatory signals (glutamate) and inhibitory signals (chemicals like gamma-aminobutyric acid, or GABA, and dopamine-related pathways) stay in balance. It is a finely tuned push-and-pull system.

In people with RLS, that balance appears to be disrupted. Brain imaging have found elevated glutamate activity in the thalamus—the brain's sensory relay station—in individuals with RLS. In other words, the brain's accelerator is being pressed too hard. Sensory signals that would normally be processed quietly are instead amplified. The nervous system is in a state of chronic overexcitation.

This explains something that has long puzzled clinicians: Why do the symptoms of RLS feel so impossible to ignore? Why does the urge to move feel so urgent, almost unbearable? It is because the brain is not just failing to send calming signals—it is simultaneously generating excessive excitatory signals. The legs are receiving a relentless "move, move, move" message that the damaged dopamine system is too depleted to counteract.

Iron connects here as well. Iron plays a role in the regulation of GABA—the brain's primary calming neurotransmitter that works in direct opposition to glutamate. When brain iron is insufficient, GABA signaling weakens. The glutamate-GABA balance tips toward overexcitation. The nervous system loses its ability to quiet itself down, particularly in the evening when other natural calming mechanisms are also at their lowest ebb.

Adenosine–The Brain's Natural Off Switch

Dopamine, iron, and glutamate form the core of the updated RLS picture—but a 2025 peer-reviewed review identified a fourth neurochemical system now understood to play a meaningful role: adenosine. This system is worth understanding because it connects the other pieces and has direct, practical implications for everyday choices.

Adenosine is a neuromodulator—a chemical that fine-tunes how neurons communicate. Think of it as the brain's built-in dimmer switch. It accumulates gradually throughout the day as a natural byproduct of neural activity, and as it builds up, it progressively dampens brain excitability and promotes the urge to rest. This is, incidentally, precisely why caffeine makes you feel more alert—caffeine works by blocking adenosine receptors, temporarily preventing that natural calming signal from getting through.

In the context of RLS, adenosine plays two important roles. First, it acts as a natural brake on overactivation—quieting sensory relay activity, reducing glutamate release, and helping the nervous system wind down toward sleep.[22] When adenosine signaling is impaired, that brake weakens, and the already overexcited RLS nervous system has even less capacity to self-calm.

Second, adenosine and dopamine receptors are physically co-located in the same movement-control brain regions—particularly the striatum. The two systems interact in a tightly coupled, opposing way: When adenosine receptors are activated, they suppress dopamine signaling; when dopamine is disrupted, the adenosine-dopamine balance tips further toward overactivation. In other words, the adenosine system and the dopamine system are not separate problems—they are interlocked, and dysfunction in one amplifies dysfunction in the other.

> *Caffeine blocks adenosine receptors—blunting the brain's natural calming system at exactly the time when the RLS-prone nervous system needs it most. For many people, this single habit is quietly making their evenings much harder than they need to be.*

This connection makes caffeine one of the more underappreciated aggravators of RLS. Even moderate caffeine consumption in the afternoon or evening can significantly blunt the body's adenosinergic wind-down process during the hours when RLS symptoms are building. Many people who cut out afternoon and evening caffeine report a meaningful reduction in symptom severity—not because caffeine is the root cause, but because removing it stops actively blocking one of the brain's key self-calming mechanisms.

The adenosine story also points toward emerging treatment possibilities. Therapies targeting adenosine receptors—particularly the A2A subtype, which has the most direct interaction with the dopamine system—are now being actively researched as potential RLS interventions.[23] For now, the most practical takeaway is this: Support your brain's adenosine system rather than suppressing it. That means managing caffeine intake thoughtfully, prioritizing consistent sleep timing, and reducing the kind of chronic stress that disrupts the nervous system's natural rhythm—all of which we will address in detail in later chapters.

Why Symptoms Peak at Night–The Circadian Iron Connection

Understanding the biology behind the evening worsening of RLS symptoms is not just intellectually satisfying—it is deeply useful for designing an effective strategy to address them.

Iron levels in the brain are not static throughout the day. They follow a circadian rhythm—a predictable daily cycle—with brain iron concentration dropping to its lowest point in the late evening and overnight hours. This is a normal biological pattern, but in people who are already working with insufficient brain iron reserves, that evening dip is enough to push the dopamine and GABA systems below the threshold needed to maintain calm, controlled movement signaling.

At the same time, dopamine naturally dips in the evening as part of the body's own preparation for sleep. For most people, this is a gentle wind-down. For someone with RLS, it means the system that is already struggling to maintain balance takes another hit precisely when they need it most.

Add to that the reduction in physical movement that comes with lying down—movement being one of the few things that temporarily resets the overactivated sensory signals—and you have the perfect conditions for an RLS flare. The body is still, the brain iron is low, dopamine is dipping, glutamate is running unchecked, and there is no movement to interrupt the cycle.

This is not bad luck. It is a predictable cascade, driven by specific biological imbalances—which means it can be predicted, planned around, and addressed.

Putting It Together—A New Way to Think About RLS

Here is the updated picture of RLS in plain terms:

- **Brain iron deficiency** is the primary upstream driver of RLS for most people. It is not always visible on routine blood tests.
- **Iron deficiency impairs dopamine regulation**—not just dopamine production, but the sensitivity of the receptors that dopamine acts on. This is why the dopamine system appears to be failing even when dopamine itself is not dramatically low.
- **Glutamate overactivity compounds the problem**, flooding the sensory system with excitatory signals that the weakened dopamine-GABA system cannot balance.
- **Adenosine dysregulation removes the brain's natural brake**, reducing the nervous system's ability to self-calm and compounding dopamine dysfunction through their shared receptor pathways.
- **The circadian iron dip triggers nightly flares**, turning marginal brain iron insufficiency into active, disruptive symptoms every evening.
- **Inflammation, gut health, and lifestyle factors** all feed into this system—either worsening the iron deficit, amplifying excitation, or both. We will address these in depth in the chapters ahead.

This framework matters because it reframes the entire approach to treatment. If dopamine dysregulation is the symptom—not the cause—then restoring dopamine with medication will always be, at best, a partial and temporary solution. The real work involves restoring the brain's iron status, calming the overactivated nervous system, and addressing the factors that are preventing the brain from getting the resources it needs.

That is exactly what the rest of this guide is designed to help you do.

Why This Changes Everything

The shift from "RLS is a dopamine problem" to "RLS is a brain iron and nervous system regulation problem" is not a minor update. It fundamentally changes what a rational, effective treatment strategy looks like.

Under the old model, the only logical intervention was to boost dopamine. Under the updated model, there are multiple meaningful points of intervention—and most of them are accessible without a prescription.

- **You can restore brain iron levels** through diet, targeted supplementation, and—in some cases—intravenous iron.
- **You can reduce inflammation** that blocks iron from reaching the brain.
- **You can calm glutamate overactivity** through specific nutrients, sleep optimization, and lifestyle adjustments.
- **You can support the GABA system**—the brain's natural brake pedal—to restore balance against excessive excitation.
- **You can protect and support the adenosine system** by managing caffeine, improving sleep consistency, and reducing the chronic nervous system overload that depletes it.
- **You can work with the circadian rhythm** rather than against it, timing interventions to match the body's predictable daily fluctuations.

None of these are experimental ideas. They are grounded in the current scientific understanding of what is actually happening in the

RLS brain—and they form the foundation of the natural strategy framework you will be working with throughout this guide.

What You Need to Take Away From This Chapter

Before we move into why conventional treatments so often fall short, lock in these core ideas:

- **Dopamine dysregulation is real in RLS**—but it is a downstream consequence, not the root cause.
- **Brain iron deficiency is the primary upstream driver**—and it may be present even when blood tests look normal.
- **Glutamate overexcitation amplifies symptoms**, turning a quiet imbalance into something that feels impossible to ignore.
- **Adenosine dysregulation removes the nervous system's natural brake**, compounding both glutamate overactivity and dopamine dysfunction—and explaining why caffeine worsens RLS.
- **The nightly timing of symptoms is predictable and biological**—driven by the circadian iron dip and evening dopamine reduction.
- This updated model opens the door to real solutions, not just symptom management.

With this foundation in place, the next step is understanding exactly why the conventional medical approach so often misses the mark—and why so many people end up more frustrated after treatment than before they started.

• • •

In Chapter 3, we examine why most conventional treatments fall short—and the specific gaps in standard testing and care that keep so many people stuck.

CHAPTER THREE

WHY MOST TREATMENTS FAIL

If you have already tried conventional treatments for RLS and found them wanting, you are not in the minority. Across the RLS community, one of the most common and deeply frustrating experiences is cycling through medications that work well at first, then stop working, or working with doctors who run tests that come back "normal" even though something is clearly wrong, or faithfully taking iron supplements for months without noticing any meaningful change.

This is not a failure of willpower or patience. It is a predictable outcome of an approach that is still catching up to the science. The conventional toolkit for RLS was built around an incomplete understanding of the condition—and the gaps in that toolkit have real consequences for the people relying on it.

This chapter walks through the four biggest ways that standard treatment approaches fall short. Understanding these gaps is not about assigning blame—it is about knowing exactly where the system is letting you down so you can make smarter, more informed decisions about your own path forward.

The Dopamine Drug Problem—Short-Term Relief, Long-Term Consequences

Dopamine agonists—medications that mimic the action of dopamine in the brain—remain among the most commonly prescribed treatments for RLS. Drugs in this category include pramipexole, ropinirole, and the rotigotine patch. For many people, they provide genuine, rapid relief. Symptoms diminish, sleep improves, and for a period of time, life feels significantly better.

The problem is what happens next.

Augmentation: When the Cure Becomes the Problem

As discussed in the previous chapter, augmentation is the phenomenon where long-term use of dopamine agonists causes RLS symptoms to intensify, spread, and become harder to control. It is not rare or obscure—it is one of the most well-documented and clinically significant problems in RLS management. Research suggests that meaningful rates of augmentation occur in people on long-term dopamine agonist therapy, with higher doses and longer duration of use associated with higher risk.

The mechanism behind augmentation tracks directly back to the science from Chapter 2. Dopamine agonists work by artificially stimulating dopamine receptors. Over time, the brain responds to this sustained artificial stimulation the way it responds to any overload: It compensates by reducing the number and sensitivity of dopamine receptors. The brain essentially turns down its own receptivity to try to restore balance. The result is that more medication is needed to achieve the same effect—and eventually, the medication that once provided relief begins to generate its own version of the problem it was meant to solve.

People experiencing augmentation often describe symptoms starting earlier in the evening, spreading to the arms or torso, occurring during the day when they never did before, and becoming more intense overall. Many assume their RLS is simply getting worse on its own—which makes sense, because that is exactly what it feels like. What is actually happening is that the treatment is driving the progression.

> *Augmentation is not a rare side effect. It is a predictable consequence of treating a downstream symptom—dopamine dysfunction—without addressing the upstream cause. The brain cannot be indefinitely fooled into calm by a system that is still starved of what it actually needs.*

Alpha-2-Delta Ligands: A Step Forward, But Still Incomplete

Partly in response to the augmentation problem, prescribing guidelines in many countries have shifted toward a different class of medications for first-line RLS treatment: alpha-2-delta ligands, which include gabapentin and pregabalin.[24] These medications work differently from dopamine agonists—they primarily calm overactive nerve signaling, which is why they also have a role in managing anxiety and certain types of pain.

For RLS, they can be genuinely helpful, particularly for people whose symptoms are driven heavily by nervous system overexcitation—the glutamate and GABA imbalance discussed in the previous chapter.

They do not carry the same augmentation risk as dopamine agonists, which is a meaningful advantage.

But they share the same fundamental limitation as every other pharmacological approach to RLS: They address symptoms without addressing the root cause. They calm the overactive nervous system without restoring the brain iron that would allow the nervous system to regulate itself. The moment the medication is reduced or stopped, the underlying imbalance is still there. For many people, symptoms return promptly and sometimes rebound.

Side effects—including dizziness, sedation, cognitive dulling, and, with pregabalin particularly, a meaningful potential for dependence—also limit how comfortably and indefinitely these medications can be used. They are not inherently wrong choices, but they are incomplete ones when used in isolation.

The Lab Testing Gap—Normal Results That Miss the Real Problem

One of the most common experiences among people with RLS is being told by a doctor that their blood work looks fine. Their hemoglobin is normal. Their serum iron is normal. Maybe their ferritin has been tested and comes back within the reference range. Case closed, presumably.

The problem, as established in Chapter 2, is that these tests are looking in the wrong place. They are measuring iron in the blood, not iron in the brain—and those are not the same thing. But even setting aside the brain-blood distinction, the standard reference ranges used to evaluate iron status are far less useful for RLS than most clinicians realize.

The Ferritin Reference Range Problem

Ferritin is the protein that stores iron in the body's tissues, and it is the single most informative iron marker for assessing RLS risk. A large and consistent body of research shows that RLS symptoms improve meaningfully when ferritin levels are raised, and that lower ferritin levels correlate with more severe symptoms—even when those levels fall within what the laboratory flags as normal.[25]

Standard laboratory reference ranges for ferritin typically start as low as 12 to 15 nanograms per milliliter (ng/mL) for adults, with the lower end of "normal" often cited around 20 to 30. The problem is that these ranges were established to identify clear iron-deficiency anemia—a condition where iron stores are so depleted that red blood cell production is compromised. They were never designed to identify the more subtle deficit in brain iron availability that drives RLS.

The research on RLS specifically points to a much higher functional threshold. Studies and clinical guidelines focused on RLS suggest that ferritin below 75 to 100 ng/mL is associated with worsening RLS symptoms, and that levels of 100 ng/mL or above appear to offer meaningful protective benefits.[26] A person with a ferritin level of 35 ng/mL would be waved through a standard blood panel without a second look—yet that level may represent a functionally significant iron insufficiency for their brain.

> *The standard ferritin reference range was built to catch anemia—not to protect the brain. A result labeled "normal" on a lab report can still represent a meaningful deficit by RLS-specific standards. Always ask for your actual number, not just whether it falls in range.*

Transferrin Saturation–The Overlooked Marker

Ferritin alone does not always tell the full story. Ferritin is an acute-phase reactant, meaning it can be artificially elevated by inflammation, infection, or liver stress—even when true iron stores are low. A person with chronic low-grade inflammation might have a ferritin reading in the 80s or 90s that looks reassuring, while their body is actually struggling to move iron into the tissues that need it.

This is where transferrin saturation becomes useful. Transferrin is the protein that transports iron through the bloodstream, and transferrin saturation reflects what percentage of that protein is actually carrying iron. A low transferrin saturation—generally below 20 percent—alongside ferritin that appears adequate can be a signal that iron transport is being impaired, not that iron stores are genuinely sufficient. In the context of RLS, low transferrin saturation may indicate that iron is not reaching the brain effectively, even if the ferritin number looks acceptable.

The practical takeaway is that a single iron marker, evaluated in isolation against a population-wide reference range, is a poor tool for assessing RLS-relevant iron status. A more useful picture requires looking at ferritin, transferrin saturation, and ideally serum iron together—and evaluating them against RLS-specific thresholds rather than anemia-prevention cutoffs.

What Gets Missed When Testing Stops at Iron

Even when iron testing is done well, it does not capture the full picture of what may be driving someone's RLS. Several other nutrient deficiencies and imbalances are meaningfully connected to RLS severity, and they are rarely tested as part of a standard workup.

- **Magnesium** plays a central role in nerve signaling and muscle relaxation. Deficiency is widespread in modern populations due to poor dietary quality and soil depletion.[27,28] Low magnesium is associated with increased nervous system excitability—which maps directly onto what we know about glutamate overactivation in RLS.[29]
- **Vitamin D** deficiency has been linked to RLS in multiple observational studies.[30] Vitamin D has broad roles in immune regulation, inflammation control, and neurological function—all relevant to the RLS picture.
- **B vitamins**—particularly folate, B6, and B12—are essential for neurological health and are known to influence RLS,[31,32,33,34] especially in pregnancy and in people with absorption issues.
- **Copper and vitamin A** are both required cofactors in the iron metabolism pathway.[35] Without adequate copper and vitamin A, the body cannot properly mobilize and utilize iron—meaning iron supplementation without addressing these cofactors may deliver limited benefit.

When none of these are tested, clinicians are working with a partial map. They may be looking at iron while the real leverage point is somewhere else entirely—or they may be addressing iron correctly while an unidentified cofactor deficiency limits how much improvement is actually possible.

The Oral Iron Problem—Why Supplements Often Disappoint

When iron deficiency is identified as a contributing factor in RLS, the standard first response is to prescribe or recommend oral iron supplements. This is a logical starting point—but it comes with limitations that are rarely explained, and those limitations go a long way toward understanding why so many people take iron for months and see little improvement in their symptoms.

The Absorption Challenge

Iron absorption from oral supplements is notoriously variable and often poor. The most commonly prescribed form—ferrous sulfate—is inexpensive and widely available, but it is also associated with significant gastrointestinal side effects including constipation, nausea, and stomach cramping. These side effects lead many people to take lower doses than prescribed, skip doses, or stop supplementing altogether.

Even when taken as directed, absorption is far from guaranteed. Iron absorption in the gut is tightly regulated by a hormone called hepcidin—and hepcidin levels rise in response to inflammation, infection, and even to iron supplementation itself. When hepcidin is elevated, it actively blocks iron from entering the bloodstream from the gut, no matter how much iron is being swallowed. Someone with chronic low-grade inflammation may be absorbing a fraction of the iron in every dose they take, regardless of how consistently they take it.

Dietary factors compound the challenge. Calcium, certain plant compounds called phytates (found in grains and legumes), polyphenols in coffee and tea, and several common medications all reduce iron absorption when consumed alongside an iron supplement.[36] Many people take their iron with morning coffee or alongside a calcium supplement without any idea that they may be significantly undermining the dose.

The Form Matters More Than Most People Know

Not all iron supplements are created equal, and the form of iron makes a meaningful difference in how well it is absorbed and how well it is tolerated. Ferrous sulfate is the most common, but it is not the best-absorbed and tends to be the most irritating to the digestive system. Ferrous bisglycinate—a form where iron is bound to the amino acid glycine—is generally better absorbed, significantly gentler on the gut, and tends to produce less of the constipation and nausea that cause people to abandon supplementation.[37,38]

Yet ferrous sulfate remains the default recommendation in most clinical settings, partly because of familiarity and partly because it is inexpensive. People who experience intolerable side effects and discontinue it are sometimes left with the impression that iron supplementation simply does not work for them—when the more accurate conclusion is that the specific form they were given was poorly matched to their physiology.

The Timeline Problem

Even when oral iron supplementation is done well—correct form, correct dose, optimal timing, no absorption blockers—the timeline for meaningful improvement is longer than most people expect. Raising ferritin levels significantly through oral supplementation typically takes several months, and raising brain iron levels may take longer still, since iron must first reach adequate levels in the blood before it can be efficiently transported across the blood-brain barrier.

Most people are not warned about this timeline. They start taking iron, check back with their doctor after four to six weeks, see modest improvement in ferritin, and are left uncertain whether to continue.

Without clear guidance about realistic timeframes and without the broader context of addressing inflammation and cofactor deficiencies simultaneously, oral iron supplementation frequently produces underwhelming results—not because it cannot work, but because it is rarely implemented with the precision and patience it requires.

> *Iron supplementation is not simply a matter of swallowing a pill. The form, timing, dose, absorption environment, and the broader inflammatory picture all determine whether that iron ever reaches the brain. Getting these details right is the difference between meaningful improvement and months of wasted effort.*

The Missing Piece–Inflammation and Gut Health

Perhaps the most significant gap in standard RLS treatment is the almost complete absence of attention to inflammation and gut health. These factors are not peripheral concerns—they sit at the center of why iron deficiency develops, why it persists, and why treatment so often stalls.

Inflammation Blocks Iron Transport

The hormone hepcidin, introduced briefly above, deserves more attention because it is so central to understanding treatment failure. Hepcidin is the body's master regulator of iron homeostasis—it is the mechanism by which the body controls how much iron enters the bloodstream and how much is stored. And hepcidin is remarkably sensitive to inflammation.

When the body detects inflammatory signals—whether from a chronic low-grade dietary pattern, gut dysfunction, excess body fat, chronic stress, overtraining, or any number of other sources—it raises hepcidin as a protective response.[39] The logic, from the body's perspective, is that bacteria and pathogens need iron to thrive, so restricting iron availability during a perceived threat is a defensive maneuver.

The problem for someone with RLS is that elevated hepcidin does not just reduce absorption of dietary iron—it also impairs the transport of iron across the blood-brain barrier. The very pathway that the brain depends on to receive the iron it needs for dopamine regulation and nerve function gets throttled. A person with chronically elevated hepcidin from persistent low-grade inflammation may never adequately restore brain iron levels regardless of how much iron they consume or supplement, because the delivery system is actively being suppressed.

This is why treating iron in isolation—without addressing the inflammatory environment that may be blocking its delivery—so often produces disappointing results. You cannot fill a tank that has a stuck valve.

The Gut-Iron Connection

Iron absorption begins in the gut, and the gut's ability to absorb iron efficiently depends on far more than simply having iron available to absorb. The integrity of the gut lining, the composition of the gut microbiome, and the degree of gut inflammation all directly influence how much iron makes it from the digestive tract into the bloodstream.

A compromised gut lining—whether from chronic stress, antibiotic overuse, highly processed diets, or conditions like irritable bowel syndrome and celiac disease—reduces the absorptive surface area available for iron uptake. Certain gut bacteria (*E. coli, S. enterica* serovar Typhimurium, *Shigella* spp., *C. jejuni*) also compete directly with the host for iron,[40] and a dysbiotic microbiome (one that is imbalanced toward less beneficial bacterial populations) can meaningfully reduce how much dietary iron is actually absorbed.[41]

Emerging research is beginning to map the specific relationship between the gut microbiome and RLS. While this science is still developing, the clinical implication is already clear: Gut health is not a separate topic from iron status. They are part of the same system. Someone addressing their iron while ignoring persistent gut dysfunction is working against themselves.

Lifestyle Factors That Quietly Worsen RLS

Standard RLS treatment rarely includes a meaningful conversation about lifestyle. Yet several everyday habits have a direct and documented impact on symptom severity—not as vague "wellness" suggestions, but through the specific mechanisms we have been discussing.

- **Chronic stress** elevates inflammatory markers, disrupts dopamine regulation, and suppresses the GABAergic calming systems that provide relief from nervous system overactivation.[42] Long-term stress is not just emotionally taxing—it is neurologically destabilizing in ways that directly worsen RLS.
- **Poor sleep** creates a vicious cycle. RLS disrupts sleep, and disrupted sleep raises inflammatory cytokines, impairs dopamine receptor sensitivity, and reduces the body's ability to restore brain iron during overnight recovery.[43] Sleep deprivation is both a consequence of RLS and an active driver of its worsening.

- **Overtraining and excessive exercise** increases iron demand significantly—the body uses iron heavily during and after intense exercise, both for oxygen delivery and for tissue repair. Athletes and highly active individuals are at elevated risk of functional iron deficiency, and excessive training without adequate nutritional recovery can deplete iron stores faster than they can be replenished.
- **A highly processed diet** is low in heme iron (from animal sources and the most bioavailable form), low in the cofactors needed for iron metabolism, high in compounds that block iron absorption, and pro-inflammatory. The modern Western dietary pattern is, in nearly every dimension, a recipe for the kind of iron insufficiency and systemic inflammation that drives RLS.

None of these lifestyle factors appear in a standard prescription pad or lab order. But their cumulative effect on the biological systems underlying RLS is as significant as any medication dose—and unlike medications, addressing them has no side effects and no augmentation risk.

The Bigger Picture–Treating Symptoms vs. Solving Problems

The thread running through all four of these treatment gaps is the same: Conventional RLS management has been built around symptom suppression rather than root cause resolution. Medications calm the signals. Labs check boxes. Supplements address deficiencies in isolation. Lifestyle is an afterthought.

None of these approaches is worthless in isolation. Medications provide real relief for real people, and there are situations where they are genuinely appropriate. Identifying and correcting iron deficiency is absolutely the right starting point. But when the pieces are deployed as standalone fixes rather than as part of a coordinated strategy that addresses the underlying biology, they consistently underperform.

What is needed is a framework—a coherent, prioritized approach that addresses the root causes in the right sequence, supports the body's own regulatory systems, and is designed to produce durable improvement rather than temporary relief.

That framework is what the rest of this guide provides.

What You Need to Take Away From This Chapter

Before moving forward, anchor these key points:

- **Dopamine medications provide real short-term relief** but carry a significant long-term risk of augmentation—a phenomenon where symptoms return worse than before, driven by the brain's compensation for chronic artificial stimulation.
- **"Normal" lab results do not rule out iron deficiency in RLS.** Standard reference ranges were designed to detect anemia, not to protect brain iron. A ferritin under 75 to 100 nanograms per milliliter may represent a clinically meaningful deficit by RLS-specific standards.
- **Oral iron supplementation is valuable but limited** by absorption challenges, form selection, inflammation, and unrealistic timelines. The form, timing, and inflammatory context all determine whether supplemental iron actually reaches the brain.
- **Inflammation—driven by diet, gut dysfunction, stress, and lifestyle—is a primary reason** iron treatment fails. Hepcidin elevation blocks iron delivery even when iron intake is adequate. Addressing inflammation is not optional; it is foundational.

- **Treating RLS effectively requires a coordinated strategy**, not a collection of isolated fixes. The next chapters build that strategy—systematically, practically, and in the right order.

• • •

In Chapter 4, we break down the full root cause picture—mapping currently known biological drivers that can fuel RLS so you know exactly what you are working with before designing your personal strategy.

CHAPTER FOUR

THE ROOT CAUSE BREAKDOWN

The previous three chapters built the conceptual foundation: what RLS is, what is actually driving it in the brain, and why conventional treatment so consistently falls short. Now it is time to get specific.

This chapter is a detailed map of currently known meaningful root cause categories that can contribute to RLS. Think of it as your diagnostic compass—not a replacement for working with a knowledgeable practitioner, but a comprehensive framework for understanding which factors may be active in your own case and why each one matters to the biology you have already learned.

Not every category will apply equally to every person. Some people reading this will have a primarily iron-driven picture. Others will find that inflammation, gut dysfunction, or specific nutrient gaps are the more prominent drivers. Many will have several categories in play simultaneously. The value of mapping all of them here is that it allows you to look at your own situation with fresh eyes and identify the factors that have been overlooked—and therefore, the levers most worth pulling.

Root Cause 1: Brain Iron Deficiency

Brain iron deficiency sits at the top of the causal chain for most people with RLS, for reasons covered in detail in Chapters 2 and 3. The assessment question here is not whether brain iron deficiency matters—it is whether it is specifically active in your case, and to what degree.

The three-marker panel most useful for this assessment is ferritin, transferrin saturation, and C-reactive protein (CRP). The targets relevant to RLS—ferritin ideally above 100 nanograms per milliliter, transferrin saturation between 25 and 35 percent, and high-sensitivity C-reactive protein (hs-CRP) low enough (ideal: < 1.0 mg/L; acceptable but concerning: 1–3 mg/L; and too high: > 3 mg/L) to confirm the ferritin level is not being artificially inflated by inflammation—are considerably more specific than standard "normal" reference ranges, and they need to be evaluated together rather than individually.

CRP is primarily used to interpret ferritin correctly, which is why hs-CRP is usually preferred—it detects low-grade inflammation which can falsely elevate ferritin. Regular CRP is like a smoke alarm that only goes off with a big fire—it's useful when inflammation is clearly high. hs-CRP is more sensitive, like a detector that can pick up even a little smoke, so it can catch low-level inflammation that still matters even when things look "normal." That's why hs-CRP is more helpful here—it ensures ferritin isn't being subtly skewed by hidden inflammation.

> *Always ask for your actual numbers, not just whether you passed. A ferritin of 32 and a ferritin of 140 are both "within range" on most lab reports—but they represent vastly different realities for your brain.*

Who Is at Elevated Risk

While brain iron insufficiency can develop in anyone, the following groups face a meaningfully higher baseline risk and should be especially vigilant about monitoring their iron markers:

- **Women of reproductive age:** Particularly those with heavy periods or low dietary meat intake, where monthly blood loss creates a persistent demand that intake rarely fully replaces.
- **Pregnant women:** The developing baby draws heavily on maternal iron stores through the second and third trimesters, which is precisely when pregnancy-related RLS rates peak.
- **Regular blood donors:** Each whole blood donation removes a meaningful amount of stored iron, and ferritin is rarely monitored between donations.
- **Endurance athletes and heavy exercisers:** iron demand during intense training is high, and distance runners face an additional loss mechanism through foot-strike hemolysis, the physical destruction of red blood cells with each footfall.
- **People following plant-based diets:** Non-heme iron from plant sources is significantly less bioavailable than heme iron from animal foods, and achieving adequate iron status without animal products requires deliberate, consistent dietary strategy.
- **People with chronic kidney disease:** Impaired iron metabolism combined with the inflammatory burden of kidney disease creates a compounded deficit that helps explain why this population has among the highest RLS rates of any group.
- **People with gastrointestinal conditions:** Any condition that damages the gut lining or impairs absorption directly depletes iron over time, regardless of dietary intake.

Root Cause 2: Inflammation Blocking Iron Transport

Hepcidin-driven inflammation—the mechanism by which chronic low-grade immune activation blocks iron from reaching the brain—was explained in detail in Chapter 3. The practical question here is whether your specific lifestyle, health history, or dietary pattern is maintaining elevated inflammation, and therefore actively preventing iron restoration even when supplementation appears adequate.

The most common drivers of the kind of smoldering, persistent inflammation that elevates hepcidin are:

- **A diet dominated by ultra-processed foods, refined seed oils, and added sugars**, which consistently elevates CRP and interleukin-6, both of which are direct hepcidin stimulators.
- **Excess visceral body fat**, which functions as metabolically active tissue that continuously releases pro-inflammatory adipokines.
- **Gut dysbiosis and intestinal permeability**, where bacterial products leak across a compromised gut lining and trigger a persistent low-level immune response.
- **Chronic psychological stress**, which sustains elevated cortisol and drives inflammatory cytokine production over time.
- **Poor or fragmented sleep**, which raises inflammatory markers and creates a direct feedback loop—RLS disrupts sleep, and disrupted sleep worsens the inflammation that is fueling the RLS.
- **Unresolved infections or active autoimmune conditions**, which keep the immune system continuously activated and hepcidin chronically elevated.

If two or more of these apply to you, there is a meaningful chance that inflammation is limiting what iron supplementation can accomplish. Addressing it is not supplementary to your strategy—it is what makes the rest of the strategy viable.

Root Cause 3: Gut Dysfunction and Absorption Failure

If ferritin levels haven't budged after months of oral iron, gut dysfunction may be why. But this is worth flagging even before supplementation begins: impaired absorption is a common and underappreciated reason iron status stays low in the first place. The following conditions and medications are among the most clinically significant absorption barriers—and several are common enough that they often go unidentified for years:

- **Proton pump inhibitors (PPIs) and antacids:** These acid-suppressing medications are among the most widely prescribed in the world, and their long-term use is consistently associated with iron deficiency because iron absorption is strongly acid-dependent.[44]
- **Undiagnosed celiac disease or non-celiac gluten sensitivity:** Iron deficiency that fails to correct with supplementation is one of the most common presenting features of undiagnosed celiac disease.[45] If you have persistent iron deficiency with no obvious cause, celiac testing is worth pursuing.
- **Inflammatory bowel disease (Crohn's and colitis):** Active gut inflammation impairs absorption while simultaneously increasing iron loss through bleeding, producing a double deficit that is very difficult to correct through oral means alone.[46]
- ***H. pylori* infection:** This extremely common stomach bacteria impairs iron absorption through multiple mechanisms and is one of the most overlooked reasons oral

iron does not raise ferritin.[47] It requires testing and treatment before iron supplementation can be expected to work.

- **Previous bariatric surgery:** Procedures that reduce stomach capacity or bypass the upper small intestine can profoundly impair iron absorption permanently,[48] often requiring IV iron rather than oral supplementation to maintain adequate levels.

Beyond these specific conditions, the gut microbiome plays a broader and still-emerging role in iron availability. Certain bacterial species actively compete with the host for dietary iron. A dysbiotic microbiome—one skewed toward less beneficial populations—can meaningfully reduce how much iron is absorbed from food or supplements, independent of any diagnosable gut condition. This is one of the reasons microbiome support through dietary diversity, fermented foods, and fiber-rich eating is an integral part of the iron restoration strategy, not a secondary consideration.

> *If you are taking iron consistently and your ferritin is barely moving, do not simply increase the dose. Ask whether your gut is actually capable of absorbing what you are already taking—the answer may be far more useful than the next pill.*

Root Cause 4: Nutrient Imbalances and Cofactor Deficiencies

Iron does not work in isolation. Its absorption, transport, storage, and utilization all depend on a network of cofactor nutrients—vitamins and minerals that must be present in adequate amounts for the iron system to function properly. Deficiencies in any of these cofactors can limit the benefit of iron restoration, amplify nervous system dysregulation, or directly worsen RLS symptoms through independent mechanisms.

Copper–The Underappreciated Iron Partner

Copper is perhaps the most important and least appreciated cofactor in iron metabolism. The enzyme ceruloplasmin—a copper-dependent protein—is essential for converting stored iron into the form that can be loaded onto transferrin and transported to the brain. Without adequate copper, iron gets trapped in storage depots and cannot be effectively mobilized, even when ferritin levels appear adequate.

This creates a paradox that traps many people: They supplement iron, ferritin climbs, but symptoms do not improve—because the iron is being stored, not delivered. Copper deficiency is a direct blocker of iron utilization. Good dietary sources of copper include beef liver, shellfish (particularly oysters), dark chocolate, nuts, and seeds. People who supplement with high-dose zinc for extended periods are particularly at risk of copper depletion, since zinc and copper compete for absorption.

Vitamin A–The Forgotten Mobilizer

Vitamin A—specifically retinol, the animal-derived form, rather than the plant-based beta-carotene precursor—plays a direct role in iron mobilization. It is required for the proper synthesis of transferrin and for promoting the release of iron from liver storage. Vitamin A deficiency impairs iron status independently of iron intake, and the two deficiencies commonly co-occur in people with poor dietary variety or significant gut absorption issues.

Liver is by far the richest combined source of both retinol and heme iron—a single serving provides meaningful amounts of both, along with copper and B vitamins. For people with RLS who can tolerate it, liver is arguably the single most targeted dietary intervention available. Even small amounts once or twice a week can make a meaningful contribution to the nutrient profile that the RLS brain needs most.

Magnesium–The Nervous System Stabilizer

Magnesium occupies a unique position in the RLS root cause map because it addresses the nervous system side of the equation rather than the iron side. It is involved in over 300 enzymatic reactions in the body, including the regulation of nerve excitability, muscle relaxation, and neurotransmitter balance—particularly the balance between glutamate and GABA.

Magnesium acts as a natural calcium channel blocker—it competes with calcium at nerve junctions and, when present in adequate amounts, reduces the rate of nerve firing. In practical terms, this means that adequate magnesium status helps buffer the kind of nervous system overexcitation that drives the restless, crawling sensations of RLS. Magnesium also directly supports GABA function, enhancing the activity of the brain's primary calming neurotransmitter.

Magnesium deficiency is extremely common—estimates suggest that a majority of adults in developed countries consume below the recommended daily amount, largely because modern food processing strips magnesium from grains and vegetables, and because chronic stress depletes magnesium through increased urinary excretion. For people with RLS, low magnesium status is not just a background deficiency—it is an active amplifier of the neurological symptoms that make RLS so disruptive.

B Vitamins—The Neurological Foundation

The B vitamin family has several members with direct relevance to RLS. Folate (B9) and B12 are both required for healthy nerve function and red blood cell production. Their deficiency is closely linked to RLS, particularly in pregnancy—where folate demand surges dramatically—and in older adults and people on long-term metformin therapy, who are at elevated risk of B12 depletion.

Vitamin B6 (pyridoxine) is a cofactor in dopamine synthesis—it is required for the enzymatic steps that convert the precursor L-DOPA into dopamine. Low B6 status can therefore impair dopamine production independently of iron status. B1 (thiamine) and B3 (niacin) support mitochondrial energy production in neurons, and deficiency in either can contribute to the kind of neurological fragility that makes RLS worse.

B vitamins work as a family, and isolated supplementation of one can sometimes mask or worsen deficiency in another. A whole-food approach to B vitamin status—centered on animal proteins, organ meats, eggs, and leafy vegetables—generally provides a more balanced and bioavailable supply than isolated supplementation.

Vitamin D—The Immune and Neurological Regulator

Multiple observational studies have found an association between vitamin D insufficiency and RLS. While a direct causal mechanism has not been definitively established, the plausible pathways are several: Vitamin D modulates inflammatory cytokine production (reducing the inflammatory drivers of hepcidin elevation), supports dopaminergic function in the brain, and plays a role in pain and sensory processing.

Vitamin D deficiency is nearly epidemic in northern latitudes and among people who spend most of their time indoors—and people with significant RLS often fall into that second category. When symptoms make evening outings unpredictable or uncomfortable, many people gradually withdraw from outside activities altogether, reducing their overall sun exposure in the process. Checking and addressing vitamin D status is a low-effort, low-risk intervention that may yield meaningful benefit as part of a broader strategy.

Root Cause 5: Lifestyle Contributors

The fifth root cause category is the one most often dismissed as too vague or too obvious to be clinically meaningful. It is neither. The lifestyle factors discussed here have documented, mechanistic connections to the neurochemical and metabolic systems underlying RLS. They are not "wellness suggestions"—they are biological inputs that either support or actively undermine everything else in your treatment strategy.

Chronic Stress–The Silent Amplifier

Chronic psychological stress dysregulates virtually every system relevant to RLS. It elevates cortisol, which over time suppresses dopaminergic function, increases inflammatory cytokine production, and disrupts sleep architecture. It activates the sympathetic nervous system—the "fight or flight" system—and keeps it chronically elevated, which works in direct opposition to the parasympathetic, rest-and-digest state that the RLS nervous system desperately needs more of.

Stress also directly depletes magnesium. When cortisol is chronically elevated, magnesium excretion through the urine increases—creating a deficiency that further destabilizes nerve regulation and amplifies the very stress response that is causing the depletion. This feedback loop is self-perpetuating, and it is one of the reasons that people going through high-stress periods so frequently report worsening RLS.

Poor Sleep—The Feedback Loop That Feeds Itself

RLS disrupts sleep, and disrupted sleep worsens RLS. This is not a metaphorical cycle—it is a biochemically precise one. Sleep deprivation raises inflammatory cytokines including interleukin-6 and TNF-alpha, both of which stimulate hepcidin production and impair iron transport. It reduces dopamine receptor sensitivity in the prefrontal cortex and striatum. It impairs the overnight restoration of brain iron that would otherwise help buffer the circadian iron dip discussed in Chapter 2.

Perhaps most importantly, poor sleep reduces the brain's adenosinergic drive the following evening. Adenosine builds up during waking hours as a natural sleep pressure signal, and it plays a key role in the gradual calming of nervous system activity toward nighttime. When sleep is disrupted and fragmented, this adenosine accumulation process is disrupted in turn—meaning the brain goes into the following evening with less of its natural calming chemical reserve.

Breaking the RLS-sleep disruption feedback loop requires addressing both ends of it—the biological drivers of RLS directly, and the sleep environment and habits that determine how restorative the sleep you do get actually is.

Overtraining–When More Exercise Becomes a Problem

Moderate, regular exercise is beneficial for RLS—it supports dopaminergic function, improves sleep quality, reduces inflammation, and can provide direct short-term relief from symptoms. But excessive training and poor recovery create the opposite effect.

Intense and prolonged exercise places enormous demands on iron. Oxygen delivery to working muscles requires iron-rich hemoglobin, and muscle repair after training requires iron-dependent enzymatic processes. Athletes and highly active individuals can deplete iron stores faster than they are replenished through diet, particularly if they are not eating sufficient animal protein and heme iron to match training demands.

High-impact exercise such as distance running also causes a phenomenon called foot-strike hemolysis—the physical destruction of red blood cells with each footfall—that adds an additional iron loss mechanism beyond what diet and supplementation typically account for.[49] For distance runners with RLS, this is a clinically meaningful factor that is almost never discussed in standard care.

The practical guidance is not to avoid exercise—it is to match training intensity and volume to recovery and nutritional capacity, and to monitor iron markers more vigilantly if exercise demands are high.

Medications That Worsen RLS

A number of commonly prescribed medications are known to either trigger or worsen RLS symptoms. Identifying whether a current medication may be contributing is an important step in the root cause assessment and is worth discussing with the prescribing clinician.

- **Antidepressants:** SSRIs (such as sertraline, fluoxetine, and escitalopram) and SNRIs are among the most commonly reported medication triggers for RLS.[50] They increase serotonin activity, which in turn suppresses dopamine pathways. Mirtazapine, a different class of antidepressant, is also strongly associated with RLS worsening.
- **Antihistamines:** Diphenhydramine, found in most over-the-counter sleep aids and allergy medications, is a dopamine antagonist that reliably worsens RLS.[51] Many people with RLS unknowingly take it to help them sleep, creating exactly the opposite of the intended effect.
- **Antinausea medications:** Metoclopramide and prochlorperazine block dopamine receptors and are well-documented RLS triggers.[52]
- **Antipsychotics:** Both older and newer antipsychotic medications block dopamine receptors and are strongly associated with inducing or worsening RLS.[53]
- **Proton pump inhibitors and antacids:** As noted earlier, these medications reduce stomach acid, impair iron absorption, and can contribute to the iron insufficiency underlying RLS over time.[54]

If any of these medications are currently part of your regimen, this information is not an instruction to stop taking them—many are prescribed for important reasons. But it is absolutely worth raising with your prescribing clinician, who may be unaware of the connection or may have an alternative available.

> *Over-the-counter sleep aids containing diphenhydramine—marketed specifically to help people sleep—are one of the most common hidden exacerbators of RLS. If you are using one of these products, stopping it may produce a faster*

> *improvement in nighttime symptoms than almost any other single intervention.*

Your Personal Root Cause Picture

Reading through these five categories, most people find that several of them resonate. That is typical. RLS rarely has a single, isolated cause—it is usually a convergence of factors, each of which individually might not be enough to tip the system into active symptoms, but together create the cumulative deficit that does.

As you review the five categories, consider which factors are most likely active in your situation:

- **Iron insufficiency**: Do you know your actual ferritin number? Is it above 100? Have transferrin saturation and CRP been checked alongside it?
- **Inflammation**: Do you have any of the common inflammatory drivers—a processed diet, excess body weight, chronic stress, poor sleep, or a known inflammatory condition?
- **Gut dysfunction**: Do you have digestive symptoms, use acid-suppressing medications, or have a history of gut conditions that could be impairing absorption?
- **Nutrient cofactors**: Is your diet consistently rich in heme iron, copper, vitamin A, magnesium, and B vitamins? Or are there gaps that may be limiting what your iron system can actually accomplish?
- **Lifestyle and medications**: Are there sleep habits, stress patterns, training loads, or current medications that may be quietly working against your progress?

Keep these questions in mind as you move into the strategy chapters. The more clearly you can identify which root causes are most active in your own case, the more precisely you will be able to apply the interventions ahead—and the faster you are likely to see meaningful results.

What You Need to Take Away From This Chapter

- **Brain iron deficiency is the primary root cause**, and ferritin above 100 nanograms per milliliter is the meaningful target—not simply "within the reference range."
- **Hepcidin-driven inflammation is the most common reason iron restoration stalls**. Addressing the sources of chronic low-grade inflammation is not optional—it is what determines whether iron treatment can actually work.
- **Gut health determines how much iron you actually absorb**. If iron supplementation has not moved your ferritin significantly, gut dysfunction is likely part of the explanation.
- **Copper, vitamin A, magnesium, B vitamins, and vitamin D** are all meaningful cofactors whose deficiency can limit progress, amplify symptoms, or both—and they are rarely assessed in standard RLS care.
- **Lifestyle factors and specific medications are not peripheral**—they have direct, documented effects on the biological systems underlying RLS, and they must be part of any serious root cause assessment.

• • •

In Chapter 5, we move from diagnosis to strategy—introducing the Restore, Deliver, and Calm framework that will guide everything that follows.

CHAPTER FIVE

THE NATURAL STRATEGY FRAMEWORK

Four chapters of science. Four chapters of understanding exactly what is happening in your body, why conventional approaches fall short, and which root causes are most likely driving your symptoms. That is not background noise—that is the foundation everything else depends on. But foundation without structure is just a pile of materials.

This chapter is where the structure arrives.

What follows is the strategic framework that organizes every practical intervention in this guide—the coherent, sequenced approach that separates a real recovery plan from a collection of disconnected supplements and habits. It is designed around three words that capture the entire logic of natural RLS management:

RESTORE

↓

DELIVER

↓

CALM

Restore iron status. Deliver iron to the brain. Calm the nervous system. Three phases—not a rigid sequence where one must be finished before the next begins, but a hierarchy of priority that mirrors the causal architecture of RLS. All three phases begin together. What the hierarchy communicates is where to invest the most weight, what to address most aggressively, and what to expect from each phase as the process unfolds. Skipping a phase, or pouring energy into Phase 3 while ignoring Phase 1, is where most natural approaches quietly fail.

Why a Framework Matters—and Why Most People Skip It

When people first realize that their RLS may have addressable root causes, the instinct to start everything at once is understandable. Order the magnesium. Look up the best iron supplement. Cut out caffeine tomorrow. Google dietary and lifestyle adjustments. Within a week, they are taking five new supplements, have completely reorganized their bedtime routine, and are watching their symptoms anxiously for any sign of change.

This approach fails—not because the individual interventions are wrong, but because without a framework they cannot build on each other. Worse, interventions deployed out of sequence can actively undermine each other. Taking high doses of iron alongside unchecked inflammation, for example, may accomplish little more than feeding the body's iron-hoarding pathways without delivering any meaningful improvement to brain iron status. Calming the nervous system with magnesium while doing nothing about the iron deficit that is destabilizing it in the first place provides temporary comfort but no forward progress.

A framework solves this. It tells you what to do, in what order, and why—so that each step you take creates the conditions for the next step to be more effective. It also prevents the discouragement that comes from doing the right things in the wrong sequence and concluding they do not work.

> *The most common reason natural approaches to RLS fail is not that they are ineffective—it is that they are deployed without a coherent sequence. The right interventions in the wrong order are still the wrong approach.*

Phase One: Restore–Building the Iron Foundation

Everything in the Restore phase is oriented around a single goal: getting iron status—specifically ferritin—into a range where the brain has the resources it needs to regulate dopamine, support GABA, and manage the neurochemical balance that keeps RLS symptoms at bay.

This is the foundation of the entire strategy. Without adequate brain iron, no amount of nervous system support will produce durable improvement. Magnesium may ease symptoms temporarily. Calming routines may improve sleep on a given night. But if the upstream iron deficit is not addressed, the system is perpetually operating below the threshold it needs to self-regulate—and every other intervention is fighting an uphill battle.

What Restore Includes

The Restore phase is primarily nutritional and supplemental. It encompasses:

- **Dietary iron optimization:** Building a consistent foundation of heme iron from animal sources, understanding which foods provide the most bioavailable iron, and learning how to pair foods to maximize absorption.

- **Intelligent iron supplementation:** Choosing the right form, timing doses correctly, avoiding absorption blockers, and understanding how to monitor progress through regular ferritin testing.
- **Cofactor nutrition:** Ensuring that copper, vitamin A, and B vitamins are present in adequate amounts so that iron can actually be mobilized and utilized, not just stored.
- **Intravenous iron (when appropriate):** For people with severe deficiency, significant absorption challenges, or RLS that has not responded to oral approaches, IV iron bypasses the gut entirely and can produce rapid, meaningful increases in ferritin. This is a medical option worth understanding even if it is not the starting point for most people.

The Restore phase is not a quick fix. Raising ferritin meaningfully through diet and oral supplementation is a process that unfolds over months, not weeks. This is one of the most important expectations to set clearly from the beginning. People who understand the timeline stay the course and see results. People who expect dramatic improvement in four weeks abandon the approach before it has had a chance to work.

Chapter 6 is dedicated entirely to the Restore phase—with specific foods, supplement forms, dosing guidance, timing strategies, and a clear picture of what progress looks like along the way.

Phase Two: Deliver—Opening the Pathway to the Brain

Restoring iron status in the body is necessary but not sufficient. The second phase addresses a question that is just as important: Once adequate iron is circulating in the blood, what ensures it actually reaches the brain?

This is where inflammation comes back to center stage. The blood-brain barrier is a highly selective gatekeeper, and the proteins responsible for transporting iron across it are suppressed when the inflammatory environment is elevated. Hepcidin, as discussed at length in the previous chapters, actively restricts iron transport under inflammatory conditions. Reducing inflammation is not just good general health advice—it is the specific mechanism by which the Deliver phase works.

Think of it in practical terms: You can spend months carefully building up your iron stores through the Restore phase, but if a chronically activated immune system is sitting at the gate blocking delivery to the brain, you are pouring iron into a pipeline with a valve that will not open. The Deliver phase is what opens the valve.

What Deliver Includes

The Deliver phase operates across three interconnected areas:

- **Anti-inflammatory nutrition:** Shifting dietary patterns away from the processed foods, refined seed oils, and added sugars that fuel systemic inflammation, and toward the whole-food, nutrient-dense patterns that support immune regulation and reduce the inflammatory signals that elevate hepcidin.
- **Targeted anti-inflammatory nutrients:** Specific compounds such as omega-3 fatty acids and polyphenols have well-documented anti-inflammatory effects and support the broader reduction in inflammatory burden that allows iron transport to normalize.
- **Gut health support:** Restoring gut lining integrity and microbiome diversity both reduces the intestinal inflammation that feeds systemic hepcidin elevation and improves the absorptive environment that determines how

much iron from the Restore phase actually enters the bloodstream in the first place.

The Deliver phase works in parallel with the Restore phase—they are not sequential steps where one must be fully completed before the other begins. Rather, they are complementary efforts that reinforce each other. Reducing inflammation while building iron status means that more of the iron being restored is actually being utilized. The two phases together are considerably more powerful than either alone.

Chapter 7 covers the Deliver phase in full—with practical dietary guidance, specific nutrient recommendations, and straightforward gut support steps that do not require a complete dietary overhaul to implement.

> *Restore and Deliver are not separate tracks—they are two hands working together. Restore builds the supply of iron the brain needs. Deliver clears the pathway so that supply can actually reach its destination. Neither works as well without the other.*

Phase Three: Calm—Quieting the Overactivated Nervous System

The third phase addresses what the first two cannot fully resolve on their own, at least not in the short term. Even as iron status improves and inflammation decreases, the nervous system does not immediately recalibrate. Glutamate overactivity has been running unchecked. The GABA system has been underpowered. Adenosine signaling has been depleted or suppressed. The brain has been stuck in a pattern of evening overexcitation, and patterns like that do not dissolve overnight.

The Calm phase is about working directly with the nervous system to accelerate that recalibration—supporting the chemical systems that inhibit overexcitation, creating the environmental and behavioral conditions that allow the nervous system to genuinely wind down in the evening, and providing the targeted quick-relief tools that make the transition period more manageable while the deeper work of Restore and Deliver takes hold.

This is also the phase that provides the most immediate, tangible relief. While Restore and Deliver are longer-game strategies whose full benefit unfolds over weeks and months, many of the Calm interventions produce noticeable results within days or even on the first night of implementation. This matters enormously for adherence—having something that works right now provides both practical relief and the motivation to stay committed to the slower foundational work.

What Calm Includes

The Calm phase is the broadest of the three, touching nutrition, targeted supplementation, daily habits, and sensory interventions:

- **Magnesium supplementation:** The cornerstone of nervous system calming for RLS. Magnesium directly supports GABA function, reduces nerve excitability, and helps buffer the glutamate overactivation that amplifies symptoms. It is the most impactful single supplement in the Calm phase for most people.
- **Nervous system regulators:** Specific amino acids including glycine and taurine support inhibitory neurotransmission, helping the brain shift into its calming mode in the evening hours when RLS is most prone to flare.
- **Targeted dopamine support:** Natural approaches to supporting dopamine signaling in the short term, including

specific botanical compounds, used strategically rather than continuously to avoid the same receptor downregulation problems that make pharmaceutical dopamine agonists problematic long-term.

- **Essential oils:** Clinically studied options that support nervous system calming, with lavender leading the evidence base. These are not merely pleasant additions—they operate through specific physiological mechanisms that are relevant to the overexcited RLS nervous system.
- **Sleep rhythm optimization:** Strategic management of light exposure, evening routine, and the behavioral conditions that allow adenosine to accumulate properly and the circadian system to work in your favor rather than against you.
- **Quick-relief tools:** A practical toolkit of fast-acting strategies for when symptoms hit acutely: movement, temperature therapy, topical magnesium, breathwork, and targeted oil application.

Chapters 8 and 9 cover the Calm phase in full, with Chapter 8 dedicated to magnesium, nervous system regulators, dopamine support, and sleep optimization, and Chapter 9 focused specifically on essential oils—including the clinical evidence for lavender, the mechanisms by which these plant compounds interact with the nervous system, and how to use them practically and effectively.

Why the Sequence Is Non-Negotiable

The hierarchy of Restore, Deliver, Calm is not arbitrary—it maps directly onto the causal chain of RLS itself. The root cause is upstream: brain iron deficiency. The bottleneck is midstream: the inflammation that blocks iron delivery. The experience is downstream: the overactivated nervous system generating symptoms every evening. Addressing the system from the top down—

not exclusively, but with appropriate weight—is what separates a strategy that produces durable resolution from one that manages symptoms indefinitely without ever resolving them.

This is why Restore and Deliver receive the most sustained investment over time, even though the Calm phase is what most people feel first.

Consider what happens when the sequence is ignored. A person who focuses exclusively on the Calm phase—taking magnesium, using essential oils, optimizing their sleep environment—may experience meaningful short-term relief. Their evenings are more manageable. They sleep better on many nights. But without Restore and Deliver running simultaneously, the underlying iron deficit continues. Over time, symptoms drift back. They conclude that magnesium stopped working, and they are not entirely wrong—but the real issue is that calming an overactivated nervous system without fixing the reason it is overactivated is a maintenance strategy, not a resolution strategy.

Conversely, a person who invests fully in Restore and Deliver but ignores Calm may find the early months genuinely difficult—because meaningful iron restoration takes time, and the nervous system does not wait patiently in the meantime. They may abandon the strategy before it has had a chance to produce results, because nothing feels different and relief is nowhere in sight.

The framework works because all three phases run in concert. Restore and Deliver address the cause. Calm addresses the experience while the cause is being corrected—and continues to play a valuable maintenance role even after iron status is optimized.

> *Think of the three phases this way: Restore is rebuilding the foundation. Deliver is clearing the*

> *construction pathway. Calm is making the building livable while the work is underway. You need all three, running simultaneously, weighted in the right order.*

Realistic Timelines—What to Expect and When

One of the most valuable things this framework can offer is honest expectation-setting. RLS did not develop overnight, and it will not resolve overnight. Understanding what a realistic timeline looks like prevents the discouragement that derails so many otherwise sound strategies.

Week One to Two—The Immediate Window

Within the first one to two weeks, the most noticeable changes tend to come from the Calm phase interventions and from removing active worseners—which is exactly what you would expect from the hierarchy. CALM addresses the downstream nervous system experience, and those interventions can shift the symptom picture quickly. RESTORE and DELIVER are running simultaneously, but their deeper work operates on a longer timeline. Stopping a dopamine-blocking medication (with appropriate medical guidance), eliminating afternoon caffeine, beginning magnesium supplementation, introducing an evening essential oil routine—these changes can produce measurable relief within days. This is the phase where many people first feel that something is genuinely shifting.

This early relief is real and meaningful. It is also not the full picture. It reflects the removal of active obstacles and the support of the nervous system's calming systems—it does not yet reflect meaningful iron restoration. Treat this early improvement as confirmation that the strategy is directionally correct, not as a signal that the deeper work can be skipped.

Weeks Four to Eight–The Foundation-Building Phase

Over the first four to eight weeks, dietary changes and iron supplementation begin to move the needle on ferritin, particularly if absorption is not severely impaired and inflammation is being meaningfully reduced. This is typically when people start noticing that the Calm phase interventions are working better and lasting longer—because the neurochemical environment is beginning to stabilize at a slightly higher baseline.

Gut support interventions also begin to show their benefit during this window, as the absorptive environment improves and more of each iron dose is actually being utilized. Anti-inflammatory dietary changes start producing measurable reductions in CRP and other inflammatory markers for many people. Progress at this stage may be subtle—fewer nights of severe disruption, slightly shorter windows of symptoms, better sleep quality overall—but it is directionally clear.

Months Three to Six–The Meaningful Improvement Window

For most people following the framework consistently, the three-to-six-month mark is where the most significant and durable improvements become apparent. Ferritin levels have moved meaningfully toward and often past the 75 to 100 nanograms per milliliter threshold. The inflammatory environment has improved. The brain's iron availability is approaching the level needed for stable dopamine and GABA function. Evening symptoms become less frequent, less intense, and more responsive to the Calm phase tools.

Some people reach a point of near-complete resolution during this window, particularly those whose RLS was primarily driven by a correctable iron deficit with limited complicating factors. Others—those with more complex pictures involving significant gut dysfunction, persistent inflammation, or more advanced iron depletion—may continue to progress through this phase more gradually. Both trajectories are normal.

Beyond Six Months—Maintenance and Optimization

Beyond the initial restoration phase, the strategy does not end—it shifts. The goal becomes maintaining the neurochemical balance that has been achieved: monitoring ferritin periodically to ensure it stays in the optimal range, continuing the dietary and lifestyle patterns that keep inflammation low, and using Calm phase tools as a maintenance layer rather than a crisis response.

Some people find that they can taper iron supplementation once ferritin is optimized and sustained through diet alone. Others find that their iron status requires ongoing supplemental support, particularly in higher-demand life circumstances. Neither outcome represents failure—individual variation in iron metabolism, absorption, and demand means that the ongoing management picture is genuinely personal.

How to Use the Rest of This Guide

The chapters that follow are organized to move through the framework in order. Each chapter is practical and specific—not a survey of possibilities but a clear, actionable guide to implementing each phase effectively.

- **Chapter 6: Restore Iron.** The complete nutrition and supplementation guide for rebuilding iron status: the best heme iron foods, vitamin C pairing, supplement forms and timing, and when intravenous iron becomes the smarter option.

- **Chapter 7: Reduce Inflammation and Deliver Iron.** The anti-inflammatory dietary strategy, key nutrients including omega-3s and polyphenols, and practical steps to support gut health and microbiome diversity.
- **Chapter 8: Calm the Nervous System.** Magnesium in depth, glycine and taurine, targeted dopamine support with *Mucuna pruriens*, sleep rhythm optimization, and adenosine-supporting habits.
- **Chapter 9: Essential Oils for RLS Relief.** The clinical evidence for lavender, mechanisms of action, application methods and blends, and the full supporting oil toolkit.
- **Chapter 10: The Practical Daily Protocol.** How all three phases integrate into a morning-to-evening daily routine that is realistic and sustainable.
- **Chapter 11: The Quick Relief Toolkit.** What to do when symptoms hit acutely, with fast-acting strategies organized for immediate use.
- **Chapter 12: When to Dig Deeper.** Signs that advanced testing or practitioner support is warranted, and how to approach that conversation with clarity.

You do not need to implement everything at once. You do not need to be perfect. What you need is a direction and a starting point—and both of those are now in hand.

What You Need to Take Away From This Chapter

- **The Restore, Deliver, Calm framework** is the organizing principle for everything that follows—a sequenced, hierarchical strategy that mirrors the actual causal architecture of RLS.
- **Restore** addresses the root—building iron status to the level the brain actually needs, through diet,

supplementation, cofactor nutrition, and when appropriate, intravenous iron.

- **Deliver** addresses the pathway—reducing the inflammation and gut dysfunction that block iron from reaching the brain, regardless of how much iron is being taken in.
- **Calm** addresses the experience—directly supporting the nervous system's ability to self-regulate through magnesium, targeted nutrients, essential oils, sleep optimization, and quick-relief tools that work while the deeper restoration is underway.
- **All three phases run simultaneously**, but with clear priorities: Restore and Deliver are the foundation; Calm is what makes the journey livable and sustainable.
- **Realistic timelines matter**. Early relief comes quickly from the Calm phase. Meaningful, durable improvement from addressing the root cause unfolds over three to six months. Expecting the former without patience for the latter is the most common reason the right approach gets abandoned.

• • •

In Chapter 6, we move into the Restore phase in full—with specific foods, supplement forms, dosing strategies, and everything you need to begin rebuilding the iron foundation your brain has been waiting for.

CHAPTER SIX

RESTORE IRON—THE FOUNDATIONAL STEP

If the previous chapters built the case for why brain iron deficiency sits at the center of RLS, this chapter is where that understanding becomes action. The Restore phase is the single most important investment you will make in this entire process—not the fastest, not the most immediately satisfying, but the most fundamentally necessary. Everything else in the strategy either supports this work or depends on it.

The goal of this chapter is practical and specific: to give you a complete, actionable guide to rebuilding iron status through the most effective combination of food, supplementation, cofactor nutrition, and—when warranted—medical iron therapy. By the end, you will know exactly what to eat, what to take, when to take it, what to avoid, and how to measure progress over time.

One framing note before we begin. Iron restoration is not a sprint. The body raises ferritin gradually—typically by a few nanograms per milliliter per month under good conditions—and brain iron availability lags behind blood markers by additional weeks.[55] This is not a reason for discouragement. It is a reason for patience and precision. Every good decision you make in this phase compounds over time. The person who implements this chapter carefully and consistently for six months will, in the large majority of cases, be living in a meaningfully different body than the one they started with.

Nutrition First–Building the Dietary Iron Foundation

Supplementation gets most of the attention in iron restoration conversations, but diet is the foundation that supplementation builds upon. A diet consistently rich in bioavailable iron does two things that supplements alone cannot: It provides iron in the form the body is best equipped to absorb and utilize, and it delivers that iron alongside the cofactors—copper, vitamin A, B vitamins, zinc—that the iron metabolism system depends on. Food is not just a delivery vehicle for iron; it is a delivery vehicle for the entire biochemical context iron needs to function.

Heme Iron–The Most Bioavailable Form

Dietary iron comes in two forms: heme iron, found exclusively in animal products, and non-heme iron, found in both plant and animal foods. The distinction matters enormously. Heme iron is absorbed at a rate of roughly 15 to 35 percent—meaning a significant proportion of what you eat actually enters your bloodstream.[56] Non-heme iron, by contrast, is absorbed at just 2 to 20 percent under the best conditions, and substantially less than that in the presence of common dietary inhibitors.[57,58] For someone working to restore depleted iron stores, this difference is not academic–it is the difference between a diet that actively builds ferritin and one that barely maintains it.

The most concentrated and bioavailable sources of heme iron, ranked by practical value for RLS recovery, are:

- **Beef liver**—the single most nutrient-dense food available for RLS recovery. A 3-ounce serving provides approximately 5 milligrams of highly bioavailable heme iron, along with substantial amounts of copper, retinol (vitamin A), B12, folate, and riboflavin. If there is one food worth introducing or increasing specifically for RLS, it is liver. Two to three servings per week makes a meaningful contribution. For those who find the taste challenging, blending small amounts into ground beef dishes or taking freeze-dried liver capsules offers a practical workaround.
- **Red meat (beef, lamb, bison)**—ground beef, steak, and other red meat cuts provide 2 to 4 milligrams of heme iron per 3-ounce serving, along with zinc, B12, and creatine. Regular red meat consumption—several times per week—forms the backbone of a dietary iron restoration strategy for most people. The concern about red meat and cardiovascular disease has been significantly overstated for unprocessed cuts,[59] and the nutrient density of quality red meat is genuinely difficult to replicate otherwise.
- **Oysters and shellfish**—shellfish, particularly oysters, are exceptional for iron restoration. A 3-ounce serving of oysters provides 4 to 7 milligrams of iron alongside the highest dietary source of zinc and meaningful amounts of copper and B12. They are worth including regularly, whether fresh, canned, or smoked.
- **Dark poultry meat**—chicken and turkey thighs and drumsticks provide more total heme iron than white breast meat (total iron: 0.9–1.1 mg per 3-ounce serving; compared to 0.3 mg per 3-ounce serving). While lower in iron than beef, they contribute meaningfully as regular dietary staples and pair well with absorption-enhancing foods.

- **Sardines and canned fish**—sardines in particular offer a practical, affordable, and well-tolerated source of heme iron (2.1–2.5 mg total iron per 3-ounce serving) with the added benefit of omega-3 fatty acids, which support the anti-inflammatory arm of the Deliver phase simultaneously.
- **Organ meats broadly**—kidney, heart, and spleen are among the most iron-dense foods available (5.4–38 mg total iron per 3-ounce serving), though they are less commonly eaten in modern Western diets. Spleen contains the highest levels, followed by kidney, and heart. Heart has a milder flavor than liver and provides a good iron-copper-B12 combination that is worth considering for those open to it.

Non-Heme Iron Sources—A Supporting Role

Plant-based iron sources—legumes, dark leafy greens, fortified grains, tofu, pumpkin seeds—have a supporting role in iron nutrition but should not be relied upon as the primary restoration strategy in someone actively trying to correct a significant deficit. Their lower bioavailability, combined with the common presence of phytates and other absorption inhibitors—known as antinutrients—in the same foods, makes them a poor foundation for rapid ferritin building.

For people following plant-based diets, this creates a genuine challenge that requires particular attention to non-heme iron optimization strategies—vitamin C pairing, soaking and fermenting legumes to reduce phytate content, and careful avoidance of competing absorption inhibitors at iron-rich meals. The supplementation section below becomes especially important in this context.

Vitamin C—The Most Powerful Absorption Enhancer

Pairing iron-rich foods—particularly non-heme sources—with vitamin C is one of the most well-supported and practically impactful strategies in dietary iron optimization.[60] Vitamin C converts iron from its less absorbable ferric form into the more absorbable ferrous form, and it counteracts the inhibitory effects of phytates and polyphenols (EGCG in green tea) on iron uptake.[61] Studies show that consuming 100 milligrams or more of vitamin C alongside a non-heme iron meal can increase iron absorption by two to four times.[62]

In practical terms, this means adding a squeeze of lemon to lentils, pairing spinach with bell pepper and citrus in a salad, or having a small glass of orange juice with an iron-containing meal. Vitamin C supplementation at mealtimes achieves the same effect and can be particularly useful for people who find it difficult to consistently include vitamin C-rich foods in iron-focused meals.

It is worth noting that vitamin C pairing matters most for non-heme iron.[63] Heme iron from animal sources is absorbed through a separate pathway that is not significantly affected by vitamin C, though there is no downside to including it.

What to Avoid at Iron-Rich Meals

Understanding what inhibits iron absorption is as important as knowing what enhances it. The following are the most impactful inhibitors to manage around iron-focused meals:

- **Coffee and tea:** Polyphenols in both beverages significantly reduce non-heme iron absorption when consumed with or shortly after a meal. Waiting 60 to 90 minutes after eating before having coffee or tea preserves a meaningful portion of the iron uptake from that meal.
- **Calcium-rich foods and calcium supplements:** Calcium competes directly with iron for intestinal absorption. Dairy products and calcium supplements should

ideally be separated from iron-rich meals or iron supplementation by at least two hours.

- **High-phytate foods:** Whole grains, legumes, and nuts consumed alongside iron sources reduce absorption. This does not mean avoiding these foods; it means being thoughtful about not pairing them with your most iron-dense meals.
- **Antacids and acid-suppressing medications:** As discussed in Chapter 4, these dramatically reduce iron absorption. If they cannot be avoided, they should be timed as far from iron intake as possible and the situation flagged for discussion with a clinician.

> *Two simple rules capture most of dietary iron optimization: Eat liver and red meat regularly, and protect your iron-rich meals by keeping coffee, tea, calcium, and antacids well separated from them. These two changes alone can significantly improve the efficiency of your dietary iron intake.*

Supplement Strategies—Getting the Most from Iron Supplementation

For most people with RLS-relevant iron deficiency, dietary iron—even as part of a well-optimized diet—will not raise ferritin to the target range quickly enough to rely on food alone. The deficit is too large, the body's iron absorption is too tightly regulated, and the timeline is too long. Strategic supplementation is the engine that accelerates what diet sets in motion.

But supplementation done poorly is barely better than not supplementing at all. The form you choose, the timing, the dose, what you take it with, and what you avoid taking it alongside all determine whether iron actually enters your bloodstream in meaningful amounts. This section covers each of those variables precisely.

Choosing the Right Form of Iron

The iron supplement marketplace is crowded, and the differences between products matter significantly. Here are the forms most relevant to RLS recovery, ranked by practical value:

- **Ferrous bisglycinate (iron bisglycinate):** The most recommended form for most people pursuing RLS-focused iron restoration. Iron is chelated to the amino acid glycine, which dramatically improves absorption—studies suggest absorption rates two to four times higher than ferrous sulfate—while producing significantly less gastrointestinal irritation.[64] It can be taken with or without food, is less affected by dietary inhibitors than ionic iron forms, and is well tolerated by the majority of people who have abandoned ferrous sulfate due to side effects. This is the form to start with.
- **Ferrous sulfate:** The most widely prescribed and least expensive form. It is effective when tolerated, but its association with constipation, nausea, and stomach cramping leads to high discontinuation rates. If cost is a significant concern and gastrointestinal tolerance is not an issue, it remains a reasonable option. Taking it with a small amount of food (rather than on an empty stomach) improves tolerance without dramatically reducing absorption.
- **Ferrous gluconate:** Gentler on the gut than ferrous sulfate and a reasonable middle-ground option, though generally considered slightly less well absorbed than ferrous bisglycinate.
- **Ferric forms (ferric citrate, ferric ammonium citrate):** Ferric iron must be converted to ferrous iron in the gut before it can be absorbed, making these forms less

efficient overall and more dependent on adequate stomach acid. They are generally not the first choice for active iron restoration.

- **Heme iron polypeptide (HIP):** Derived from animal hemoglobin and absorbed through the same highly efficient pathway as dietary heme iron. Well tolerated, less susceptible to inhibitors, and effective, but considerably more expensive than other oral options. Worth considering for people who have not responded adequately to non-heme supplement forms.
- **Liposomal iron:** Iron encapsulated in a lipid layer that protects it from gut irritation and bypasses some of the standard absorption regulation pathways. An emerging option with promising tolerability data, particularly for people with sensitive digestive systems or inflammatory gut conditions (an absorption-impaired state).

Dosing–How Much and How Often

Iron supplementation dosing has been substantially revised in recent years based on emerging research into how the body regulates iron absorption. The old approach—high daily doses to maximize iron intake—turns out to be counterproductive.[65] When iron is taken at high doses every day, hepcidin spikes in response to each dose and remains elevated the following morning, actively blocking absorption of the next day's dose. You end up in a cycle where each dose partially defeats the one that follows.

The current evidence-based approach is alternate-day dosing: taking iron every other day rather than every day. This strategy allows hepcidin to return to baseline between doses, meaning each dose is absorbed in a more favorable hormonal environment. Research comparing daily and alternate-day dosing consistently shows that total iron absorbed is similar or even higher with alternate-day dosing, with reduced gastrointestinal side effects.[66]

A typical starting dose for iron restoration in RLS is 25 to 65 milligrams of elemental iron per dose, taken on alternate days. Ferrous bisglycinate supplements are often labeled by their total weight rather than elemental iron content—check the label carefully. They generally contain about twenty percent elemental iron, meaning 65 mg of ferrous bisglycinate provides about 13 mg of elemental iron and you would need to take two servings to reach the lower end of the starting dosage range. The elemental iron content is what matters, not the total weight of the compound.

For people with more severe deficiency or consistently poor absorption, doses toward the higher end of this range or once-daily dosing may be warranted—but this is best guided by regular ferritin monitoring and, ideally, clinical input rather than independent escalation.

Timing–When to Take Iron for Maximum Absorption

Timing iron supplementation correctly can meaningfully increase how much is absorbed from each dose. The key principles:

- **Take iron on an empty stomach when possible:** Absorption is highest when the stomach is empty and acid levels are elevated. This typically means first thing in the morning, before breakfast, or at least one to two hours after a meal.
- **Pair with vitamin C:** Taking 100 to 250 milligrams of vitamin C alongside an iron supplement boosts absorption of non-heme iron forms and has no downside. A small glass of orange juice, a vitamin C supplement, or 100 milligrams of ascorbic acid all work.

- **Morning timing has an additional advantage:** Hepcidin is naturally lower in the morning hours, meaning the absorption environment is more favorable earlier in the day than later.

- **Separate from calcium, coffee, tea, and other supplements by two hours**: This includes multivitamins containing calcium or zinc, which compete with iron for absorption.

- **Separate from magnesium supplements:** Iron and magnesium compete for absorption pathways. Take them at different times of day—iron in the morning, magnesium in the evening is an arrangement that works well for both.

> *The single most impactful change most people can make to their iron supplementation protocol is switching from daily to alternate-day dosing. If you have been taking iron every day without meaningful improvement in ferritin, this change alone—combined with the right form and timing—often produces the progress that has been missing.*

Monitoring Progress–Ferritin Testing and What to Look For

Iron supplementation without regular monitoring is like navigating to an unfamiliar place without GPS. You need to know whether your strategy is working, how quickly, and when you have reached the target range. Ferritin testing—along with transferrin saturation and ideally CRP—should be repeated every eight to twelve weeks during active iron restoration.

A meaningful response to oral supplementation is generally considered a rise of at least 10 to 15 nanograms per milliliter per month under good absorption conditions.[67] If ferritin is rising but slowly, the strategy may need refinement—form, timing, or absorption environment. If ferritin is not rising despite consistent supplementation, gut dysfunction, hepcidin elevation from inflammation, or a competing absorption blocker is almost certainly involved, and the Deliver phase interventions need to be prioritized more aggressively.

The target is ferritin at or above 100 nanograms per milliliter, with 100 to 150 being the range where most people with RLS begin to notice meaningful, durable symptom improvement. Once this range is achieved, testing every three to four months is sufficient to ensure levels are being maintained.

When to Consider Intravenous Iron

For most people, oral supplementation combined with dietary optimization is the right starting point. But for a meaningful subset—those with severe deficiency, significant gut absorption challenges, or RLS that has been unresponsive to well-implemented oral strategies—intravenous (IV) iron is a genuine option that deserves to be understood rather than dismissed as an extreme measure.

Why IV Iron Is Different—and Sometimes Necessary

Intravenous iron bypasses the gut entirely. It delivers iron directly into the bloodstream in doses that would be impossible to achieve through any oral approach, and it does so in a single session or a short series of infusions rather than over months of daily supplementation. Hepcidin regulation, gut absorption variability, and dietary inhibitors become irrelevant—the iron is in the blood and ready to be transported.

The clinical evidence for IV iron in RLS is strong. Multiple randomized controlled trials have shown that intravenous iron sucrose and ferric carboxymaltose—the two most commonly used IV iron formulations for RLS—produce significant improvements in symptom severity, sleep quality, and quality of life.[68,69,70] Some meta-analyses and reviews have concluded that ferric carboxymaltose is superior for IV iron administration. The benefit appears to be durable in many patients, with some studies showing maintained improvement for twelve months or more following a single infusion course.

An important practical question for anyone considering IV iron is whether it needs to be repeated. The answer is that it depends on the underlying cause of the iron deficit. If the deficit was primarily situational—a pregnancy, a period of heavy blood loss, a temporary dietary gap—a single course of IV iron may be sufficient to restore ferritin durably, particularly when combined with ongoing dietary optimization. If the deficit reflects a chronic pattern—persistent poor absorption, ongoing high iron demand from exercise or menstrual loss, or continuing inflammatory iron blockade—ferritin will gradually drift downward again after IV iron, and periodic re-treatment is likely necessary. This is not a failure of the approach; it simply reflects the ongoing management reality of a chronic condition.

Who Is a Strong Candidate for IV Iron

The following situations represent particularly strong indications for considering IV iron rather than continuing with oral supplementation:

- **Ferritin remains below 50 nanograms per milliliter** despite three to four months of well-implemented oral iron supplementation with correct form and timing.
- **Confirmed gut absorption impairment**—celiac disease, inflammatory bowel disease, post-bariatric surgery, or other documented absorptive conditions that make oral restoration fundamentally limited.
- **Severe, daily RLS symptoms** with significant quality of life impairment, where the months-long timeline for oral restoration is causing serious harm and faster improvement is medically justified.
- **Intolerance to all well-absorbed oral iron forms** despite trying gentler formulations and optimized timing.
- **RLS in the context of kidney disease or dialysis**—where oral iron is typically ineffective due to the compounded iron metabolism disruption of kidney disease, and IV iron is already standard practice in many nephrology settings.

Having the Conversation with Your Clinician

IV iron is a prescription treatment that requires a clinician's involvement, and it is not uniformly available through primary care. Neurologists and sleep medicine specialists familiar with RLS are more likely to be aware of the evidence base than general practitioners who may have limited familiarity with the RLS-specific iron research.

Going into that conversation prepared makes a significant difference. Bringing documented ferritin levels, a record of oral supplementation attempts and their outcomes, and a clear articulation of symptom severity and its quality-of-life impact gives the clinician the information needed to make a well-informed referral decision. If the first conversation is not productive, a second opinion from a specialist with RLS expertise is entirely reasonable.

IV iron is generally safe and well-tolerated. Mild reactions—flushing, temporary muscle aches, a brief dip in phosphate levels—can occur in some people but are manageable and transient. Serious adverse reactions are rare with modern IV iron formulations and appropriate pre-screening.

Cofactor Nutrition—Making Sure Iron Can Do Its Job

Restoring iron status is not just about getting iron in—it is about ensuring the body has everything it needs to actually use that iron. Two cofactors are so critical to iron metabolism that they deserve specific attention in the Restore phase: copper and vitamin A. Without both of them present in adequate amounts, iron supplementation may raise ferritin while delivering limited benefit to brain iron availability.

Copper—Ensuring Iron Moves Out of Storage

As discussed in Chapter 4, the copper-dependent enzyme ceruloplasmin is required to convert stored iron into the form that can be loaded onto transferrin for transport to the brain. Without adequate copper, iron accumulates in storage but cannot be mobilized and delivered. This is one of the most commonly overlooked reasons for poor response to iron supplementation—ferritin may even rise, indicating iron is being stored, while transferrin saturation remains low because the stored iron is not being released.

Copper supplementation is not something to approach casually—excess copper creates its own problems, and the balance between copper and zinc is delicate. The most sensible approach for most people is to ensure dietary copper is adequate through food rather than relying primarily on supplementation. The best dietary sources of copper are beef liver (exceptional), oysters, dark chocolate (at least 70 percent cocoa), cashews, and sunflower seeds. Liver, again, stands out as the most practical combined source of iron, copper, and vitamin A simultaneously.

People who supplement with high-dose zinc—a common practice in immune or testosterone support protocols—are at particular risk of copper depletion, since zinc and copper compete for intestinal absorption. Many consider a supplemental ratio of 10:1 to 15:1 zinc to copper to be ideal, meaning for every 10–15 mg of zinc you should supplement 1 mg of copper. If you are supplementing with more than 15 to 20 milligrams of zinc daily on a regular basis, copper status deserves attention.

Vitamin A–The Iron Mobilization Partner

Retinol—the animal-sourced form of vitamin A—plays a direct role in iron mobilization by promoting transferrin synthesis and stimulating the release of iron from hepatic (liver) storage. Vitamin A and iron deficiencies commonly co-occur, and correcting iron without addressing vitamin A insufficiency can significantly blunt the expected response.

An important distinction: The beta-carotene found in orange and yellow vegetables is a precursor to vitamin A but converts to retinol inefficiently in many people, particularly those with certain genetic variants, hypothyroidism, or gut dysfunction.[71] Relying on beta-carotene from plants as a substitute for retinol is a common error in plant-forward diets. True retinol comes from animal sources—liver, egg yolks, full-fat dairy—and liver provides the most concentrated and bioavailable supply available.

If dietary liver is not a regular part of your eating pattern, it is worth considering either introducing it in small amounts or exploring a high-quality cod liver oil supplement, which provides both retinol and vitamin D in their most bioavailable forms.

Putting the Restore Phase Together—A Practical Starting Point

The Restore phase does not require a complete dietary overhaul or a complex supplementation protocol. It requires a handful of consistent, well-executed practices applied with appropriate patience. Here is a practical starting framework:

- **Eat red meat at least three times per week**, with liver included once or twice. If liver is not palatable, freeze-dried liver capsules are an acceptable alternative.
- **Begin iron supplementation with ferrous bisglycinate**, 25 to 65 milligrams of elemental iron, on alternate mornings before breakfast, paired with 100 to 250 milligrams of vitamin C.
- **Separate iron from coffee, tea, calcium, magnesium, and zinc** by at least two hours. Taking iron first thing in the morning (before coffee or tea, and away from a calcium-containing breakfast) and reserving magnesium for the evening naturally handles the iron-magnesium conflict. The harder discipline for most people is the coffee and tea window: if your morning routine moves straight from waking to caffeine, consider taking iron immediately upon waking and waiting at least two hours before your first cup.
- **Protect iron-rich meals by having coffee and tea before the meal**, not during or immediately after.

- **Include oysters, sardines, or other shellfish regularly** for copper, zinc, and additional iron—several times per month at minimum.
- **Test ferritin, transferrin saturation, and CRP every eight to twelve weeks** and track progress over time. Know your numbers. Adjust based on results, not assumptions.
- **If ferritin does not move meaningfully after twelve weeks**, prioritize the Deliver phase interventions more aggressively—the pipeline may be blocked by inflammation or gut dysfunction rather than insufficient iron intake—and discuss IV iron options with a knowledgeable clinician.

> *Ferritin is the scorecard of the Restore phase. Everything in this chapter is aimed at moving that number toward and past 100 nanograms per milliliter—and keeping it there. Test it, track it, and let it guide your adjustments. It is the most objective feedback available on whether this phase is working.*

What You Need to Take Away From This Chapter

- **Heme iron from animal foods—particularly liver, red meat, and shellfish—is the most bioavailable dietary iron source** and forms the irreplaceable foundation of the Restore phase.
- **Ferrous bisglycinate is the preferred supplemental iron form** for most people—better absorbed and better tolerated than the widely prescribed ferrous sulfate.
- **Alternate-day dosing outperforms daily dosing** by allowing hepcidin to return to baseline between doses, improving net absorption with fewer side effects.
- **Timing, pairing, and separation matter as much as dose**. Morning dosing on an empty stomach with vitamin C and away from absorption inhibitors can significantly multiply the effectiveness of each supplement dose.

- **Copper and vitamin A are essential cofactors** that determine whether stored iron is mobilized and delivered—liver provides both in the most bioavailable form available.
- **IV iron is a legitimate and evidence-supported option** for those with severe deficiency, absorption failure, or inadequate response to oral strategies—not a last resort, but a well-timed tool.
- **Ferritin testing every eight to twelve weeks is essential** for tracking progress and making informed adjustments. The target is 100 nanograms per milliliter or above.

• • •

In Chapter 7, we turn to the Deliver phase—addressing the inflammation and gut dysfunction that determine whether the iron you are restoring actually reaches the brain where it is needed most.

CHAPTER SEVEN

REDUCE INFLAMMATION—UNLOCKING IRON DELIVERY TO THE BRAIN

Imagine spending months carefully rebuilding your iron stores through everything in Chapter 6—consistent dietary changes, well-timed supplementation, regular testing—only to find that your ferritin is climbing while your RLS symptoms are barely budging. It is more common than it should be, and it is almost always explained by the same overlooked variable: inflammation.

Iron is only half the equation. The other half is delivery—ensuring that the iron circulating in your blood actually crosses the blood-brain barrier and reaches the brain regions that need it most. As established in earlier chapters, this delivery process is actively regulated by hepcidin, and hepcidin is acutely sensitive to inflammatory signals. A chronically inflamed system is a system with a partially closed gate—and no amount of iron on the outside of a closed gate makes any difference to what is happening on the inside.

This chapter is the Deliver phase in full—a practical guide to reducing the inflammatory burden that blocks iron transport, supporting the gut systems that determine how much iron enters the bloodstream in the first place, and equipping the body with the specific nutritional tools most relevant to both. None of this requires a radical lifestyle overhaul. It requires understanding which levers matter most—and pulling them consistently.

The Anti-Inflammatory Dietary Foundation

Diet is the most powerful lever available for shifting the body's inflammatory baseline. Not because food is medicine in the simplistic sense, but because the inflammatory signaling pathways that elevate hepcidin and impair iron delivery are directly fueled or suppressed by what you eat every day. Chronic dietary patterns that favor whole, minimally processed foods consistently produce lower levels of inflammatory markers—C-reactive protein, interleukin-6, TNF-alpha—than patterns dominated by processed and refined foods. The mechanism is not mysterious; it is biochemistry responding to inputs.

The goal of the anti-inflammatory dietary foundation is not perfection—it is a meaningful net shift in the daily inputs that either feed or dampen the inflammatory signals driving hepcidin elevation. Small, consistent changes in the right direction produce more lasting benefit than short-term dietary perfection followed by a return to previous patterns.

The Case Against Ultra-Processed Foods

Ultra-processed foods—the packaged, shelf-stable, industrially manufactured products that now constitute a significant proportion of caloric intake in most Western countries—are among the most potent dietary drivers of chronic inflammation. They are high in refined carbohydrates that spike insulin and promote glycation, high in added sugars that generate oxidative stress, and rich in industrially refined seed oils that provide an unbalanced excess of omega-6 fatty acids.

The omega-6 issue deserves particular attention in the RLS context. Omega-6 and omega-3 fatty acids compete for the same enzymatic pathways in the body, and the balance between them determines whether those pathways produce pro-inflammatory or anti-inflammatory signaling molecules. In traditional dietary patterns, the ratio of omega-6 to omega-3 intake was roughly 4:1 or lower. In the modern Western diet, driven largely by the widespread use of refined vegetable and seed oils in processed foods, that ratio has climbed to 15:1 or higher in many people. This imbalance chronically biases the body toward inflammatory signaling—not dramatically, but persistently, in the same low-grade way that elevates hepcidin and slowly undermines iron delivery over months and years.

Reducing ultra-processed food intake does not require calorie counting or elaborate meal planning. The most practical approach is a simple displacement strategy: Replace processed food staples one category at a time with whole-food alternatives. Packaged snacks replaced with nuts or fruit. Refined grain products replaced with root vegetables or legumes. Seed oil-based condiments replaced with olive oil or butter. Each substitution does not need to be perfect—what matters is the cumulative direction of change over time.

Seed Oils–A Specific Target

Refined seed oils—canola, soybean, corn, sunflower, safflower, and cottonseed oils—deserve specific attention because they are so ubiquitous in the modern food environment that most people consume them in quantities they are entirely unaware of. These oils are the primary fat source in nearly all fast food, most restaurant cooking, the vast majority of packaged foods, and many products marketed as healthy alternatives.

The problem is their extraordinarily high omega-6 content, primarily in the form of linoleic acid, and the oxidative instability of polyunsaturated fats when exposed to the high heat of industrial processing and cooking. Oxidized lipids are particularly potent inflammatory triggers. Reducing seed oil consumption—by cooking at home with more stable fats like olive oil, butter, ghee, or coconut oil, and by reducing restaurant and processed food intake—is one of the highest-leverage dietary changes available for shifting the inflammatory baseline.

The popular claim that seed oils drive inflammation deserves a closer look. Current evidence does not show that higher linoleic acid intake from seed oils increases common inflammatory markers in healthy people; so the blanket condemnation of seed oils as inherently inflammatory is not well supported. The more legitimate concern is what happens to these oils before and during cooking. Seed oils are rich in polyunsaturated fats that oxidize readily under high heat or prolonged storage, and oxidized lipid products can act as inflammatory signaling molecules.[72] The issue, in other words, is less about the oil itself and more about how it has been handled, processed, and heated. Many people also report feeling better when they reduce seed oil consumption, which is worth taking seriously even where the mechanistic picture remains incomplete.

What to Build Toward—The Anti-Inflammatory Plate

Rather than framing this as a list of foods to avoid, it is more useful to describe what an anti-inflammatory dietary pattern actually looks like in practice:

- **Animal proteins as the foundation:** Red meat, poultry, eggs, and fish provide heme iron, omega-3s (particularly in fatty fish), and the complete amino acid profiles that support tissue repair and immune regulation. These are the backbone of both the Restore and Deliver phases simultaneously. While fish is primarily known for delivering omega-3s and red meat protein and minerals, grass-fed beef can meaningfully contribute to a healthy omega-6-to-omega-3 ratio. It has a omega-6:omega-3 ratio of between 1.5:1 and 3:1 (compared to grain-fed beef at 7:1 to 15:1). Lamb and bison meat have a ratio of roughly 2:1.
- **Fatty fish two to three times per week:** Salmon, mackerel, sardines, anchovies, and herring are the richest dietary sources of long-chain omega-3 fatty acids (EPA and DHA), which are the most potent dietary anti-inflammatory agents available. This single dietary change, sustained over eight to twelve weeks, produces measurable reductions in CRP and other inflammatory markers in most people.
- **Colorful vegetables in abundance:** Deeply colored vegetables—dark leafy greens, brassicas, beets, red onions, bell peppers, berries—are rich in polyphenols, carotenoids, and other plant compounds with documented anti-inflammatory properties. They also provide fiber that feeds the beneficial gut bacteria central to the gut health component of this chapter.
- **Olive oil as the primary cooking and dressing fat:** Extra-virgin olive oil is the most well-researched anti-inflammatory dietary fat. Its oleocanthal content produces anti-inflammatory effects through similar pathways to ibuprofen, and its polyphenol profile supports both vascular health and gut microbiome diversity.[73]
- **Whole food carbohydrates rather than refined ones:** Root vegetables, legumes, and whole fruits provide fiber, micronutrients, and a lower glycemic impact than refined grains and added sugars. They feed beneficial gut bacteria

without the inflammatory signaling associated with rapid blood sugar spikes.

> *The anti-inflammatory dietary shift does not require a label—Mediterranean, ancestral, whole food, or otherwise. It requires a practical move in one direction: more whole foods, fewer processed ones, with fatty fish and olive oil as consistent anchors. Pursued consistently over weeks and months, this shift measurably reduces the inflammatory environment that is keeping the gate to your brain's iron supply partially closed.*

Key Anti-Inflammatory Nutrients—Targeted Support Beyond the Diet

Dietary patterns set the foundation, but specific nutrients—whether from food or targeted supplementation—can provide concentrated anti-inflammatory support that meaningfully accelerates the Deliver phase. The following are the most evidence-supported options for reducing inflammation in the specific context of RLS recovery.

Omega-3 Fatty Acids—The Anti-Inflammatory Cornerstone

Omega-3 fatty acids—specifically eicosapentaenoic acid (EPA) and docosahexaenoic acid (DHA) from marine sources—are the most robustly researched anti-inflammatory nutritional intervention available. They work by competing with omega-6 arachidonic acid for the enzymes that produce eicosanoids, shifting production away from pro-inflammatory prostaglandins and leukotrienes toward anti-inflammatory and pro-resolving mediators called resolvins and protectins.

In practical terms, adequate EPA and DHA intake helps dampen the chronic low-grade inflammatory signaling that elevates hepcidin and impairs iron transport to the brain. Studies on omega-3 supplementation consistently show reductions in CRP, IL-6, and TNF-alpha over eight to twelve weeks of consistent use—precisely the inflammatory markers most relevant to hepcidin regulation.[74]

DHA also has direct neurological relevance beyond its anti-inflammatory effects. It is a structural component of brain cell membranes and is concentrated in the dopaminergic regions of the brain most affected in RLS. Adequate DHA status is associated with better dopamine receptor sensitivity and more efficient synaptic signaling—a benefit that complements the iron restoration work of the Restore phase.

For dietary sources, fatty fish two to three times per week provides meaningful EPA and DHA. For supplementation, a fish oil or algae-based omega-3 supplement providing a combined 1,000 to 2,000 milligrams of EPA plus DHA (not the total fish oil in the serving, but the actual DHA and EPA) daily is a practical and well-tolerated approach for most people. Quality matters—choose products that have been third-party tested for oxidation and purity and come in triglyceride form, and store them in the refrigerator after opening to minimize lipid oxidation.

Vitamin D—Immune Regulation and Neurological Support

Vitamin D is less a nutrient in the conventional sense and more a steroid hormone that regulates the expression of hundreds of genes—including many involved in immune function and inflammatory signaling. Vitamin D receptors are found throughout the immune system, and vitamin D insufficiency consistently predicts higher levels of inflammatory cytokines in observational research. From the Deliver phase perspective, addressing vitamin D deficiency is relevant to reducing the inflammatory drivers of hepcidin elevation.

From the neurological perspective, vitamin D receptors are also present in dopaminergic brain regions, including the substantia nigra—the same region showing iron deficiency in RLS imaging studies.[75] Animal research suggests that vitamin D supports the maintenance and function of dopaminergic neurons.[76] While the direct causal evidence in humans is not yet definitive, the convergence of anti-inflammatory and neurological relevance makes vitamin D insufficiency a priority target in RLS recovery.

Vitamin D status is best assessed by a 25-hydroxyvitamin D blood test. A level of 40 to 60 nanograms per milliliter (ng/mL) is a widely recommended baseline for general health—many laboratory reference ranges use a lower threshold of 30, which reflects minimum sufficiency rather than optimal function. An ideal level usually falls in the range of 50–80 ng/mL. For people testing below 40, supplementation with 5, 000 IU (and up to 10,000 IU under the guidance of a clinician) of vitamin D3 daily is a reasonable starting point, taken with a meal containing fat for optimal absorption. Vitamin K2 (50 to 200 mcg) is a useful cofactor to take alongside vitamin D3 for people supplementing at higher doses, as it supports proper calcium metabolism.

Polyphenols–Plant Compounds with Measurable Anti-Inflammatory Effects

Polyphenols are a broad family of plant compounds that include flavonoids, anthocyanins, resveratrol, quercetin, and hundreds of related molecules. They are responsible for much of the color in deeply pigmented fruits and vegetables, and they have multiple mechanisms of anti-inflammatory action—including inhibition of the NF-kB pathway, a central regulator of inflammatory gene expression, and direct antioxidant activity that reduces the oxidative stress that feeds inflammatory signaling.[77]

The most practical and evidence-supported polyphenol sources for regular dietary inclusion are:

- **Berries:** Blueberries, blackberries, cherries, and strawberries are among the richest polyphenol sources available and have demonstrated anti-inflammatory effects in clinical research.[78] Fresh, frozen, or unsweetened dried forms all provide meaningful polyphenol content.
- **Extra-virgin olive oil:** Beyond its fatty acid profile, olive oil provides oleocanthal, hydroxytyrosol, and oleuropein—polyphenols with potent anti-inflammatory activity that distinguish extra-virgin from refined olive oils. The distinctive peppery throat sensation from high-quality extra-virgin olive oil is oleocanthal in action.
- **Dark chocolate and cocoa:** At 70 percent cocoa content or above, dark chocolate is a meaningful source of flavonoids with anti-inflammatory and vascular benefits.[79] It also provides copper, relevant to the Restore phase cofactor discussion. Two to three squares daily is a practical and enjoyable way to include it.
- **Green tea:** Rich in epigallocatechin gallate (EGCG), green tea one of the most studied polyphenols for anti-

inflammatory effects. One practical consideration: Green tea contains compounds that inhibit iron absorption. Drink it well away from iron-rich meals and iron supplementation—two to three hours of separation is sufficient.

- **Red onions, apples, and capers:** Among the richest dietary sources of quercetin, a flavonoid with well-documented anti-inflammatory and antihistamine properties. Regular inclusion in cooking is an easy way to build consistent polyphenol diversity.

Curcumin–Targeted Anti-Inflammatory Support

Curcumin—one of the active compounds in turmeric—is one of the most extensively studied botanical anti-inflammatory agents. It works through multiple mechanisms, most notably through inhibition of the NF-kB pathway and suppression of COX-2 enzyme activity—the same pathway targeted by common anti-inflammatory medications, but through a gentler, broader mechanism without the gastrointestinal risks of prolonged NSAID use.[80]

The primary challenge with curcumin is bioavailability—standard turmeric powder is poorly absorbed on its own. Several formulations have been developed to address this, with the most practical options being curcumin combined with piperine (the active compound in black pepper, which increases curcumin absorption by up to 2,000 percent) or phospholipid-complexed curcumin (such as Meriva or BCM-95), which substantially improves absorption without requiring piperine. Other better, but less available options include curcumin combined with turmeric essential oil and turmeric combined with fenugreek fiber (CurQfen).

A dose of 500 to 1,000 milligrams of a bioavailable curcumin formulation daily has shown anti-inflammatory benefit in clinical research. It is best taken with food containing fat, which further supports absorption. Culinary turmeric in cooking provides some benefit and is worth including as a dietary practice, but therapeutic anti-inflammatory effects typically require a well-absorbed supplement formulation rather than relying on food amounts alone.

One note of caution: Curcumin and certain polyphenols may reduce iron absorption if taken at the same time as iron-rich foods or iron supplements. As with green tea, a two-hour separation from iron intake is a sensible precaution.

Gut Health Support—Restoring the Foundation of Iron Absorption

The gut is where iron enters the body and where a significant proportion of the inflammatory signaling driving hepcidin elevation originates. Supporting gut health is therefore not a separate concern from iron delivery—it is integral to it. A gut that absorbs iron inefficiently and generates chronic low-grade inflammation is an environment actively working against the Restore phase. A gut that absorbs well and maintains a healthy mucosal barrier is one of the most powerful enablers of iron delivery available.

The good news is that meaningful improvement in gut function does not require extreme dietary restrictions, expensive testing, or prolonged protocols. A relatively small number of consistent practices produce the majority of the benefit.

Feed the Microbiome—Fiber as the Foundation

The gut microbiome thrives on fermentable dietary fiber—the kind found in vegetables, fruits, legumes, and whole grains. Beneficial bacterial species ferment this fiber to produce short-chain fatty acids

(SCFAs), particularly butyrate, propionate, and acetate. Butyrate is the primary fuel source for the cells lining the gut wall, and adequate butyrate production is one of the most important determinants of gut lining integrity. A gut lining that is well-maintained by butyrate-producing bacteria is one that absorbs iron efficiently and generates less inflammatory leakage into the systemic circulation.

Increasing dietary fiber diversity—rather than simply fiber quantity—is the most effective strategy for enriching microbiome diversity. Aiming for 30 or more different plant foods per week has emerged as a practical benchmark associated with microbiome richness in research settings. This does not mean large amounts of any individual food; it means variety. A handful of different vegetables, a rotation of legumes, seeds mixed into meals, seasonal fruit—the cumulative variety matters more than any single high-fiber food.

Fermented Foods—Probiotic Support Through Diet

Fermented foods introduce live beneficial bacteria directly into the gut and provide additional short-chain organic acids that support a healthy gut environment. Research comparing fermented food intake to high-fiber diets has found that fermented foods produce a more rapid and measurable increase in microbiome diversity—making them a particularly efficient tool for gut microbiome support.[81]

The most practical and evidence-supported fermented foods for regular inclusion are:

- **Plain, full-fat yogurt**—one of the most accessible and well-tolerated fermented foods, rich in *Lactobacillus* and *Bifidobacterium* species with substantial research support. Choose unsweetened varieties to avoid the inflammatory effects of added sugar.

- **Kefir**—fermented milk with a broader probiotic diversity than most yogurts. Dairy-based kefir is the most well-studied, but water kefir provides a non-dairy alternative for those who do not tolerate dairy.
- **Sauerkraut and kimchi**—lacto-fermented vegetables that are among the richest dietary sources of live bacteria. Choose refrigerated, unpasteurized versions—pasteurized sauerkraut has been heat-treated and no longer contains live cultures. A small serving (a few tablespoons) with a meal is sufficient for meaningful benefit.
- **Miso and tempeh**—fermented soy products that provide both probiotic organisms and prebiotic fiber. Miso in soup form is a particularly simple way to incorporate fermented foods into a regular eating pattern. Note: the vast majority of soybeans are genetically modified, so look for organic and non-GMO labels.

Probiotic Supplementation–When Food Is Not Enough

For people with significant gut dysfunction, a history of antibiotic use, or difficulty consistently including fermented foods in their diet, a probiotic supplement provides a reliable way to introduce beneficial bacterial species. The evidence base for specific probiotic strains in the direct treatment of RLS is limited, but the indirect case through gut barrier integrity and inflammation reduction is well-supported.

A multi-strain probiotic containing a combination of *Lactobacillus* and *Bifidobacterium* species, at a dose of 10 to 100 billion CFU daily, is a reasonable starting point. Strains with the most research support for gut barrier function and inflammation reduction include *Lactobacillus rhamnosus GG*, *Lactobacillus plantarum*, *Bifidobacterium longum*, and *Bifidobacterium infantis*.[82] Pairing a probiotic supplement with prebiotic fiber from food maximizes its benefit by ensuring the introduced bacteria have adequate substrate to survive and colonize.

Supporting the Gut Lining—Healing What Has Been Compromised

For people with evidence of gut lining compromise—indicated by digestive symptoms, food sensitivities, a history of gut conditions, or significant antibiotic exposure—specific interventions to support mucosal healing are a meaningful addition to the Deliver phase. The most evidence-supported options are:

- **L-glutamine:** The primary fuel source for intestinal epithelial cells. Supplemental L-glutamine at doses of 5 to 10 grams daily has been shown to support gut barrier integrity and reduce intestinal permeability in clinical research. It is well tolerated, inexpensive, and mixes easily into water or smoothies. Take the powder form on an empty stomach, preferably first thing in the morning.
- **Bone broth:** Rich in glycine, proline, and hydroxyproline—amino acids that support the structural integrity of the gut mucosal layer. Regular bone broth consumption is one of the most traditional and nutritionally coherent gut support strategies available, and it also provides small amounts of minerals including iron.
- **Zinc carnosine:** A chelated zinc compound with specific evidence for supporting gut lining repair and reducing intestinal inflammation. At a dose of 75 milligrams daily, it has demonstrated benefits for mucosal integrity in clinical trials.[83] Note that ongoing zinc supplementation requires monitoring copper status, as discussed in Chapter 6.
- **Reducing unnecessary antibiotic exposure:** Each course of broad-spectrum antibiotics causes significant

disruption to the microbiome that can take months to partially recover. This is not a recommendation to avoid antibiotics when they are genuinely needed, but a reminder that the risk-benefit calculation is worth discussing explicitly with a clinician for ambiguous cases such as sinusitis, mild ear infections, or upper respiratory tract infections where antibiotics may provide marginal benefit.

> *Gut health and iron delivery are not separate topics—they are the same topic viewed from different angles. A healthy gut lining absorbs more iron from the Restore phase. A diverse microbiome reduces the gut-derived inflammation that elevates hepcidin. Investing in gut health is simultaneously investing in every other part of the strategy.*

Stress, Sleep, and Lifestyle–The Non-Dietary Drivers of Inflammation

Diet and targeted nutrients do the heavy lifting in the Deliver phase, but two non-dietary factors contribute meaningfully to the inflammatory burden that blocks iron delivery: chronic stress and insufficient sleep. Both have direct, documented effects on the inflammatory markers most relevant to hepcidin elevation, and both are often more addressable than people assume.

Chronic Stress–Reducing the Inflammatory Load

The relationship between chronic psychological stress and inflammatory signaling is well-established. Sustained cortisol elevation—the hormonal hallmark of chronic stress—upregulates NF-kB pathway activity, the same pathway that many anti-inflammatory dietary interventions are targeting.[84] It also directly increases interleukin-6 and CRP over time. From the Deliver phase perspective, failing to address significant chronic stress while aggressively pursuing anti-inflammatory nutrition is working with one hand tied behind your back.

Stress reduction strategies with the most documented effects on inflammatory markers include regular moderate aerobic exercise (20 to 40 minutes three to five times per week reduces CRP meaningfully over eight to twelve weeks),[85] mindfulness-based practices including meditation and slow diaphragmatic breathing (which downregulate sympathetic nervous system activity and reduce cortisol),[86] spending consistent time in natural environments,[87] and ensuring adequate social connection—loneliness is an independent predictor of elevated inflammatory markers with an effect size comparable to many dietary interventions.[88]

None of these need to be dramatic interventions. A daily 20-minute walk in a natural setting, consistent slow breathing practice in the evening, and one or two sessions of meaningful social connection per week produce measurable changes in the body's inflammatory tone over time. The consistency matters more than the intensity.

Sleep–Protecting the Anti-Inflammatory Nighttime Window

Sleep is the body's primary anti-inflammatory maintenance window.[89] Deep, restorative sleep suppresses inflammatory cytokine production, allows the gut lining to repair, and restores the hormonal balance that keeps hepcidin regulation functioning properly. Disrupting this window—due to RLS itself, poor sleep hygiene, or environmental factors—sustains the inflammatory environment that is blocking iron delivery.

Protecting sleep quality during the Deliver phase should be a priority, not an afterthought. The Calm phase chapter covers sleep optimization in detail, but even before that—removing electronic screens from the bedroom, maintaining a consistent sleep and wake time, keeping the sleeping environment cool and dark, and avoiding alcohol (which fragments sleep architecture even when it initially promotes sleep onset) are changes that directly reduce the inflammatory consequences of disrupted sleep. Don't forget to diffuse calming and sleep-supportive essential oils like lavender, Roman chamomile, vetiver, and cedarwood.

Putting the Deliver Phase Together—A Practical Starting Framework

Like the Restore phase, the Deliver phase works through consistent daily practice rather than dramatic intervention. Here is a practical starting framework that captures the most impactful elements without requiring a complete life reorganization:

Daily Non-Negotiables

- **Replace seed oils in home cooking** with olive oil, butter, ghee, or coconut oil. This single change, sustained consistently, produces one of the most meaningful reductions in daily pro-inflammatory input available without changing what you eat.
- **Include fatty fish at least twice per week**—salmon, sardines, or mackerel. On other days, a high-quality fish oil supplement providing 1,000 to 2,000 milligrams of combined EPA and DHA covers the remainder.
- **Add a fermented food to at least one meal daily**—a tablespoon of sauerkraut, a serving of plain yogurt, or a cup of kefir. This does not need to be elaborate or expensive.

- **Prioritize vegetable variety over quantity**—rotate through different colors and types over the course of a week rather than eating large amounts of one or two favorites.

Supplement Starting Points

- **Omega-3 (if dietary fish intake is below twice weekly):** 1,000 to 2,000 milligrams EPA plus DHA daily, from a third-party-tested fish oil or algae oil supplement.
- **Vitamin D3:** 2,000 to 5,000 IU daily with a fat-containing meal, adjusted based on 25-hydroxyvitamin D testing. Pair with K2 (50–200 micrograms MK-7) if supplementing above 2,000 IU regularly.
- **Curcumin (for those with elevated CRP or known inflammatory conditions):** 500 to 1,000 milligrams of a bioavailable formulation (with piperine or phospholipid complex) daily with a meal containing fat. Separate from iron supplementation by two hours.
- **Probiotic (if fermented food intake is limited or gut symptoms are present):** a multi-strain Lactobacillus and Bifidobacterium product at 10 to 50 billion CFU, taken with food.

How to Know the Deliver Phase Is Working

The clearest objective signal that the Deliver phase is producing results is a rising transferrin saturation alongside rising ferritin. If ferritin is climbing but transferrin saturation remains stubbornly below 20 percent, inflammation is still impairing iron transport and the Deliver phase interventions need to be intensified. If both markers are rising together, iron is being absorbed and transported—the gate is opening.

Subjectively, the early signs that inflammation is decreasing include improved energy levels and morning vitality, better mood stability, reduced digestive symptoms, and—over time—evenings that feel somewhat less fraught than they did before. These improvements often precede the full benefit of ferritin normalization, because reducing inflammation directly reduces neurological overexcitation in its own right, independent of the iron delivery benefit.

Testing CRP alongside the iron panel every eight to twelve weeks provides the most useful picture of Deliver phase progress. A CRP declining from elevated toward below 1 milligram per liter confirms that the inflammatory burden driving hepcidin elevation is being meaningfully reduced.

What You Need to Take Away From This Chapter

- **Inflammation is the primary reason iron restoration stalls**. Elevated hepcidin from chronic low-grade inflammation blocks iron transport to the brain regardless of how much iron is being taken in. The Deliver phase directly addresses this blockade.
- **Reducing ultra-processed foods and refined seed oils** is the highest-leverage dietary change for shifting the inflammatory baseline—not because of any single component, but because of the cumulative pro-inflammatory burden they represent.
- **Omega-3 fatty acids, vitamin D, polyphenols, and curcumin** are the most evidence-supported targeted nutrients for reducing the inflammatory markers most relevant to hepcidin regulation and iron delivery.
- **Gut health is integral to both iron absorption and systemic inflammation**. Fermented foods, dietary fiber diversity, and—where needed—L-glutamine and targeted probiotic supplementation are the most practical gut support interventions.

- **Chronic stress and disrupted sleep sustain inflammation independently of diet.** Addressing both—even partially—meaningfully reinforces the dietary and nutritional work of this chapter.
- **Rising transferrin saturation alongside rising ferritin is the objective signal** that the Deliver phase is working. Tracking both markers together every eight to twelve weeks provides the clearest picture of whether iron's pathway to the brain is opening.

• • •

In Chapter 8, we move into the Calm phase—the nervous system interventions that provide immediate, tangible relief while the foundational work of Restore and Deliver unfolds over time.

CHAPTER EIGHT

CALM THE NERVOUS SYSTEM—IMMEDIATE RELIEF AND LASTING BALANCE

The Restore and Deliver phases address the root of RLS—the brain iron deficit and the inflammatory environment that sustains it. But those phases operate on a timeline measured in weeks and months. In the meantime, you still have to get through tonight. And tomorrow night. And the night after that.

That is where the Calm phase earns its place. While Restore and Deliver are rebuilding the neurochemical foundation, Calm works directly with the nervous system as it is right now—not the nervous system you will have in three months, but the one that is overactivated every evening, running short on GABA, flooded with glutamate, and sending relentless movement signals down to your legs. The goal is not to mask those signals permanently with medication. It is to give the nervous system the specific resources and conditions it needs to begin regulating itself—and to make each night genuinely more manageable while the deeper work proceeds.

This chapter covers four interconnected areas of nervous system support: magnesium, the most impactful single intervention for most people; targeted calming amino acids that directly support inhibitory neurotransmission; strategic dopamine support for acute symptom management; and sleep rhythm optimization that works with the brain's own biology rather than fighting it. Together, they form the practical toolkit that makes RLS livable while the foundational work unfolds.

Magnesium—The Cornerstone of Nervous System Calm

Of all the nutritional interventions in the Calm phase, magnesium stands alone in terms of the breadth of its nervous system relevance and the immediacy with which it can produce noticeable results. It is the mineral the overactivated RLS nervous system is most likely to be short on—and it addresses the neurochemical imbalance underlying RLS symptoms through multiple simultaneous mechanisms.

Magnesium's role in nervous system regulation is grounded in three interconnected mechanisms. First, it acts as a natural blocker of NMDA receptors—the receptors that glutamate binds to in order to excite neurons.[90] Magnesium physically sits inside the NMDA receptor channel and blocks it when the channel is at rest, only allowing excitatory signals through when a neuron is sufficiently active to warrant it. When magnesium is deficient, this blocking mechanism weakens and NMDA receptors become abnormally responsive—a state of hypersensitivity that maps almost exactly onto the glutamate overexcitation picture described in Chapter 2.

Second, magnesium directly supports GABA-A receptor function—the primary receptor through which the brain's main calming neurotransmitter acts.[91] Adequate magnesium facilitates the conformational (specific three-dimensional shape or structure of a receptor protein) changes that allow GABA-A receptors to respond effectively to GABA, enhancing the inhibitory signaling that counterbalances glutamate overactivity. In essence, magnesium simultaneously reduces excitatory signaling and boosts the sensitivity of calming signaling—addressing both sides of the excitation-inhibition imbalance that characterizes RLS.

Third, magnesium is required for the activation of more than 300 enzymes throughout the body, including those involved in ATP energy production in neurons, muscle relaxation, and the synthesis of serotonin—which in turn is the precursor to melatonin, the primary sleep-onset signal.[92] Low magnesium therefore ripples through the entire neurological and metabolic infrastructure that supports calm, restorative sleep.

Why Magnesium Deficiency Is So Common

Magnesium deficiency is not a niche problem. Surveys consistently show that a majority of adults in developed countries consume below the recommended daily amount—roughly 400 milligrams for men and 310 milligrams for women.[93,94,95] The reasons are structural. Modern food processing strips magnesium from grains during refining. Industrial agriculture has gradually depleted magnesium content from soils, reducing it in vegetables even when those vegetables are eaten regularly. Refined sugars and alcohol accelerate urinary magnesium excretion. And chronic stress—through elevated cortisol—drives magnesium out of cells and into urine, creating a self-reinforcing loop in which the stress that worsens RLS simultaneously depletes the mineral most needed to buffer it.

Standard blood tests measure serum magnesium—the magnesium circulating in blood plasma—which represents less than one percent of total body magnesium.[96] The vast majority is stored in bones and soft tissues. Serum magnesium can appear normal while intracellular and tissue magnesium stores are substantially depleted, meaning that a normal blood test does not meaningfully rule out functional magnesium deficiency. If symptoms suggest deficiency, therapeutic trial of supplementation is more informative than waiting for a blood test to confirm it.

Choosing the Right Magnesium Form

Not all magnesium supplements are equivalent. The form determines both how well the magnesium is absorbed from the gut and, in some cases, which tissues it preferentially reaches. Here are the most relevant forms for RLS management:

- **Magnesium glycinate (bisglycinate):** The recommended starting form for most people with RLS. Magnesium chelated to the amino acid glycine is well absorbed, highly bioavailable, and gentle on the digestive system. Critically for RLS, glycine itself is an inhibitory neurotransmitter with calming properties—meaning magnesium glycinate provides a dual nervous system benefit that other forms do not. It is the best-tolerated form and the most appropriate for consistent daily use.
- **Magnesium threonate (L-threonate)**: A newer form specifically developed for neurological applications. Magnesium threonate has demonstrated superior ability to cross the blood-brain barrier and raise brain magnesium concentrations compared to other forms, in both animal studies and early human research.[97] For people primarily seeking neurological and cognitive benefits—which is the central goal in RLS—this form has a compelling advantage.

It is more expensive than other options but worth considering for those who have not achieved adequate symptom relief with glycinate.

- **Magnesium malate:** Magnesium bound to malic acid, which plays a role in the cellular energy cycle—is well absorbed and generally well tolerated. A reasonable alternative for those who find glycinate less effective, and may be particularly appropriate for people experiencing significant daytime fatigue alongside their RLS.
- **Magnesium citrate**: One of the more commonly available forms, reasonably well absorbed, and significantly less expensive than glycinate or threonate. The main limitation is that at higher doses it tends to have a laxative effect, which can become limiting for people trying to take therapeutically meaningful amounts. Useful at lower doses or as a budget option, but not the first choice for RLS-focused supplementation.
- **Magnesium oxide:** The most common form found in low-cost supplements and multivitamins. Its bioavailability is poor—only around four percent is absorbed in most studies.[98] Despite being labeled with a high milligram content, it delivers far less usable magnesium than any of the chelated forms at lower doses. It is worth checking whether a current magnesium supplement is in this form before concluding that supplementation is not working.
- **Topical magnesium (magnesium chloride flakes or oil):** Applied directly to the legs as a lotion, spray, or bath soak. While research on transdermal magnesium absorption is less robust than for oral forms, many people with RLS report meaningful symptom relief from topical magnesium applied to the legs before bed—possibly through local muscle relaxation effects as much as systemic absorption. It is a useful complement to oral supplementation rather than a replacement, and is particularly practical as a quick-relief tool when symptoms are actively flaring.

Dosing and Timing Strategies

A therapeutic starting dose for magnesium supplementation in RLS is 200 to 400 milligrams of elemental magnesium daily, from a well-absorbed form such as glycinate or threonate. The elemental magnesium content—not the total weight of the compound—is the relevant number. Many magnesium glycinate products, for example, are sold as 400-milligram capsules containing only 80 milligrams of elemental magnesium. Reading labels carefully prevents inadvertent underdosing.

Timing matters significantly. The most relevant window for RLS management is the evening—specifically one to two hours before the time symptoms typically begin. This positioning allows magnesium to be absorbed and reach peak tissue levels during the highest-risk period of the night. A split dose—a smaller amount in the morning and the larger portion in the evening—can help build overall tissue levels while still concentrating the calming benefit in the evening hours.

For people who have been severely deficient for a prolonged period, meaningful saturation of tissue stores can take four to six weeks of consistent supplementation before full neurological benefits are realized. A lack of immediate dramatic effect in the first week is not a signal to abandon the approach—consistent daily use is what builds the tissue reserve that produces lasting change.

As noted in Chapter 6, magnesium and iron compete for absorption pathways and should be taken at different times. Morning iron, evening magnesium is the arrangement that serves both goals optimally without either undermining the other.

> *Magnesium glycinate in the evening is the single most commonly reported effective natural intervention for*

> *RLS among people who have explored the full landscape of options. If only one supplemental change is made in the Calm phase, this is the one to make—at the right dose, in the right form, at the right time of day.*

Nervous System Regulators—Glycine and Taurine

Beyond magnesium, two amino acids have direct and well-documented roles in calming nervous system overactivation in ways that are specifically relevant to the RLS picture: glycine and taurine. Both work through the inhibitory neurotransmitter systems that are underactive in RLS, and both are safe, well-tolerated, and practically easy to use.

Glycine—The Inhibitory Amino Acid

Glycine is both a structural protein building block and a functional inhibitory neurotransmitter in its own right. In the spinal cord and brainstem, glycine receptors mediate inhibitory signaling that helps regulate motor neuron activity—the very neural pathways involved in the movement-related symptoms of RLS. Glycine also inhibits NMDA glutamate receptors through a co-agonist binding site, providing an additional mechanism of glutamate dampening that complements magnesium's NMDA-blocking action.

In sleep research, glycine supplementation before bed has demonstrated the ability to improve sleep quality and reduce the time to reach slow-wave sleep—the deepest and most restorative stage—without causing morning grogginess.[99,100] This makes it particularly valuable for the RLS context, where the goal is not simply to induce sleep by sedation but to create the neurological conditions in which sleep can proceed naturally and restoratively.

A practical dose of glycine for sleep and nervous system support is 3 to 5 grams taken 30 to 60 minutes before bed. Glycine powder dissolves easily in water and has a pleasant, mildly sweet taste—making it one of the most user-friendly supplements in the Calm phase toolkit. It is worth noting that magnesium glycinate provides both magnesium and glycine simultaneously, meaning people taking this form of magnesium are already receiving some glycine benefit—though additional targeted glycine supplementation can provide a larger dose than what is bound in the magnesium compound.

Taurine—The Calm Beneath the Storm

Taurine is a sulfur-containing amino acid found in high concentrations in the brain, heart, and skeletal muscle. Despite its reputation from energy drink marketing—where it is listed as an ingredient alongside stimulants, creating a misleading association—taurine itself is profoundly calming. It acts as a GABA-A receptor agonist, directly activating the brain's primary inhibitory receptor system, and it modulates glycine receptors in the brainstem and spinal cord.[101] In animal models, taurine consistently reduces excitatory neurological activity and demonstrates anticonvulsant and anxiolytic (anxiety-relieving) effects.[102]

In the RLS context, taurine's primary value is its ability to enhance inhibitory tone—essentially giving the brain's braking system a more reliable grip. It also supports magnesium retention within cells, meaning it complements magnesium supplementation by helping maintain the intracellular magnesium concentrations that nervous system regulation depends on.

A practical dose for nervous system support is 500 milligrams to 2 grams taken in the evening, 30 to 60 minutes before bed. It combines well with glycine—the two can be taken together and their mechanisms of action are complementary rather than overlapping. Taurine is generally well tolerated, and side effects at these doses are uncommon.

> *Glycine and taurine together form a simple, low-cost evening protocol that supports inhibitory neurotransmission through multiple pathways simultaneously. Think of them as turning up the volume on the brain's own calming system at exactly the time of night when RLS is working hardest to override it.*

Targeted Dopamine Support—*Mucuna Pruriens* as a Strategic Tool

One of the most common questions among people exploring natural approaches to RLS is whether there is a natural way to support dopamine signaling—one that provides some of the relief associated with pharmaceutical dopamine medications without carrying the augmentation risk that makes those medications so problematic long-term.

The most clinically relevant natural option in this area is *Mucuna pruriens*—a tropical legume whose seeds contain significant concentrations of L-DOPA, the direct biochemical precursor to dopamine. L-DOPA is also the pharmaceutical form of dopamine precursor therapy used in Parkinson's disease treatment, but in Mucuna it exists within a whole-plant matrix that appears to modulate its pharmacological activity differently than isolated pharmaceutical L-DOPA.[103]

How Mucuna Pruriens Works in RLS

When *Mucuna pruriens* is consumed, the L-DOPA in the seed crosses the blood-brain barrier and is converted to dopamine by the enzyme aromatic amino acid decarboxylase—the same step that vitamin B6 facilitates, which is why adequate B6 status supports this conversion. The resulting increase in dopamine availability can temporarily relieve the dopaminergic signaling deficiency that contributes to evening RLS symptoms.

Several small clinical studies have examined *Mucuna pruriens* in the context of Parkinson's disease, and the results suggest that the whole-plant extract produces a smoother, more sustained dopamine effect with less of the peak-and-crash profile associated with pharmaceutical L-DOPA.[104] Whether this advantage fully translates to the RLS context has not been studied in rigorous controlled trials, but the mechanistic logic is sound and the clinical experience among RLS-focused practitioners is broadly positive for short-term and strategic use.

When Mucuna May Help

Mucuna pruriens is most likely to be useful in two specific RLS scenarios:

- **Evening symptoms that are interfering significantly with sleep onset**—taken 30 to 60 minutes before the typical onset of symptoms, Mucuna can reduce the severity and urgency of the evening RLS window during the period before Restore and Deliver interventions have had time to produce meaningful neurochemical improvement.
- **Acute bridging support during the early weeks of the strategy**—the three-to-six-month timeline for meaningful iron restoration means there is an early period

when the foundational work is underway but symptoms have not yet improved substantially. Mucuna used strategically during this window can make that period significantly more manageable without committing to the dopamine agonist escalation cycle.

Critical Considerations—Use Strategically, Not Daily

Mucuna pruriens is a meaningful tool, but it carries the same fundamental cautions as any intervention that works by increasing dopamine signaling. The difference between Mucuna and pharmaceutical dopamine agonists is one of degree and mechanism, not of kind.

- **It can lose effectiveness over time:** Chronic daily use may lead to receptor downregulation similar to, though likely milder than, what occurs with pharmaceutical dopamine agonists.[105] This is the most important reason to use it strategically rather than as a permanent daily supplement.
- **It may worsen symptoms if overused:** The augmentation-like rebound that characterizes long-term pharmaceutical dopamine therapy may occur with Mucuna as well, particularly with high doses taken every day over extended periods. Using the minimum effective dose, with regular days off, significantly reduces this risk.
- **It is best used occasionally or in defined windows:** A few nights per week rather than nightly, or during particularly high-demand periods such as travel, significant life stress, or the early weeks of the iron restoration strategy. Once ferritin and iron delivery are approaching the target range and the nervous system is better supported by magnesium and the Calm phase tools, the need for Mucuna typically diminishes naturally.

- **Avoid combining with pharmaceutical dopamine medications:** Mucuna contains L-DOPA and should not be used alongside prescription dopaminergic drugs without explicit guidance from the prescribing clinician, as combining dopamine-raising interventions can produce unpredictable effects.

A starting dose of 100 to 300 milligrams of a standardized Mucuna pruriens extract (typically standardized to 15 percent L-DOPA content) taken 30 to 60 minutes before the symptom onset window is a reasonable starting point. Begin at the lower end and titrate—gradually adjust the dose to the optimal amount that provides therapeutic effect and minimizes side effects—upward based on effect and tolerance. Products should clearly state their L-DOPA content by percentage so that dosing can be calibrated accurately.

> *Mucuna pruriens is a bridge, not a destination. It provides meaningful symptomatic support during the window before the foundational work takes full effect. Used strategically and sparingly—never daily long-term—it can make the early months of recovery substantially more tolerable without creating the receptor downregulation problems that make pharmaceutical dopamine agonists so problematic.*

Sleep Rhythm Support—Working With the Brain's Own Timing System

The neurochemical interventions covered above—magnesium, glycine, taurine, and targeted dopamine support—address what is happening inside the brain. But what happens around the brain matters almost as much. The environment and behaviors in the hours before sleep either support or actively undermine the delicate neurochemical conditions those supplements are working to create.

The brain's sleep system has two primary drives: the adenosine-mediated sleep pressure that builds throughout the day (discussed in Chapter 2), and the circadian rhythm that times alertness and drowsiness according to light and darkness. RLS disrupts both. The adenosine system is compromised by caffeine, stress, and fragmented sleep. The circadian system is disrupted by artificial light exposure, irregular schedules, and stimulating evening activities. Aligning behavior with these systems—rather than fighting them—is one of the most effective and underutilized strategies in RLS management.

Light Exposure—The Circadian Anchor

Light is the primary signal that sets and maintains the circadian clock. Morning bright light exposure—ideally natural sunlight, but a broad-spectrum light therapy lamp works well in low-light seasons or climates—is one of the most powerful tools for anchoring the circadian system and establishing a consistent biological day. Exposure within the first hour of waking, for at least 10 to 20 minutes, sets in motion the hormonal cascade that will, approximately 14 to 16 hours later, produce the melatonin surge that drives sleep onset.

The evening counterpart is equally important. The human eye contains specialized photoreceptors—intrinsically photosensitive retinal ganglion cells containing the photopigment melanopsin—that are extraordinarily sensitive to blue-wavelength light. These receptors send signals directly to the suprachiasmatic nucleus, the brain's master circadian clock, suppressing melatonin production in response to light that resembles daylight. Modern artificial lighting, particularly LED screens and energy-efficient lighting, is heavily blue-enriched and capable of significantly suppressing melatonin production when encountered in the two to three hours before bed.

The practical implications are clear and specific. In the evening hours, shifting to warmer, dimmer lighting reduces the circadian disruption from artificial light. Blue-light-blocking glasses—amber-tinted lenses that filter short-wavelength light—provide a practical solution for people who cannot avoid screens in the evening. Most modern devices also offer night mode or warm color shift settings that reduce blue light emission after sunset. These are not trivial adjustments—research consistently shows that they measurably improve melatonin onset timing and sleep quality,[106] and they are particularly relevant for the RLS nervous system that is already fighting an uphill battle to settle in the evening.

Caffeine—Revisiting the Adenosine Connection

Chapter 2 established the neurochemical basis for caffeine's impact on RLS through the adenosine system. This is the place to translate that understanding into practical timing guidance.

Caffeine has a half-life of approximately five to seven hours in most adults—meaning that a cup of coffee consumed at 2 p.m. still has half of its adenosine-blocking effect active at 7 to 9 p.m. For someone whose RLS symptoms typically begin around 9 or 10 p.m., afternoon caffeine is directly blunting the adenosine accumulation that should be helping the nervous system wind down during precisely that window.

The evidence-based recommendation is to avoid caffeine after noon for people with RLS. This can feel dramatic for people accustomed to afternoon coffee, but the neurological benefit is substantial. For those who find a hard noon cutoff difficult, a gradual shift—pushing the last caffeine dose earlier by 30 minutes every few days—achieves the same end point with less disruption to daily routine. Green tea, matcha, and caffeinated soda, while lower in caffeine than coffee, still block adenosine receptors and fall under the same guidance.

The Evening Wind-Down Routine—Building Biological Permission to Rest

The brain does not transition abruptly from alert to asleep—it needs a graduated transition period during which physiological arousal decreases, body temperature begins to drop, and the neurochemical environment shifts toward the inhibitory dominance that sleep requires. For people with RLS, this transition is already compromised by the biological factors covered throughout this guide. A deliberate evening routine creates the behavioral conditions that support the transition rather than impeding it.

A practical wind-down routine for RLS does not need to be elaborate or rigid. What matters is consistency and direction—a reliable signal to the nervous system that the day is ending and the conditions for rest are being assembled. The following elements represent the most impactful building blocks:

- **Dim the environment 90 to 120 minutes before bed:** Shift from overhead lighting to lamps, candles, or other low-level warm light sources. This is one of the simplest and highest-impact changes available for melatonin onset timing.
- **Take evening supplements during the wind-down window:** Magnesium glycinate, glycine, taurine, and any Mucuna dose should be timed to the wind-down routine

rather than taken immediately at bedtime. This gives supplements time to be absorbed and reach peak effect during the high-risk symptom window.

- **Reduce cognitive and emotional stimulation:** News, emotionally engaging social media, and work-related thinking all maintain sympathetic nervous system activation. Replacing them in the final 60 to 90 minutes before bed with low-arousal activities—reading physical books, light stretching, conversation with a partner, listening to calm music—reduces the cortisol and noradrenaline that work against the calming transition.
- **Cool the sleeping environment:** Core body temperature must drop by approximately one to two degrees Fahrenheit to initiate and maintain sleep. A cooler bedroom (roughly 65 to 68 degrees Fahrenheit or 18 to 20 degrees Celsius) supports this drop. For people who run warm or live in warmer climates, a cooling mattress pad or lightweight, breathable bedding makes a meaningful difference.
- **Apply essential oils during the wind-down:** Topical or diffused lavender and other calming oils, covered in detail in the next chapter, integrate naturally into the wind-down window and provide an additional sensory anchor for the calming transition.
- **Maintain consistent sleep and wake times:** The circadian system is a clock, and clocks need regularity to keep accurate time. Irregular sleep schedules prevent the circadian system from building the reliable patterns of melatonin onset and cortisol suppression that facilitate smooth sleep onset. Even a 30-minute consistency window—going to bed within 30 minutes of the same time every night, including weekends—produces measurable improvements in sleep quality over two to four weeks.

Breathwork—The Nervous System's Emergency Brake

Breathwork is perhaps the most underestimated tool in the RLS Calm phase toolkit—not because it is subtle, but because its effects are immediate, reliable, and available at zero cost at any moment of the day or night. Slow, diaphragmatic breathing directly activates the vagus nerve, shifting the autonomic nervous system from sympathetic (fight-or-flight) to parasympathetic (rest-and-digest) dominance. This shift reduces cortisol, lowers heart rate, and—critically for RLS—reduces the sympathetic overactivation that amplifies sensory overexcitation in the evening.

Two specific breathing patterns have the strongest evidence base for nervous system calming:

- **4-7-8 breathing.** Inhale through the nose for a count of four, hold for a count of seven, exhale slowly through the mouth for a count of eight. The extended exhale relative to the inhale is the key—it stimulates the vagus nerve more potently than shorter exhales. Repeat four to six cycles. This pattern is particularly effective when symptoms are building and the urge to move is intensifying.
- **Box breathing (equal-count breathing).** Inhale for a count of four, hold for four, exhale for four, hold for four. Repeat for four to six cycles. Slightly less potent than 4-7-8 for acute calming but easier for beginners and equally effective for the evening wind-down routine when practiced before symptoms peak.

Integrating two to five minutes of intentional breathwork into the wind-down routine—before symptoms have peaked—is more effective than deploying it reactively after they have already become intense. Like all Calm phase tools, breathwork delivers its greatest benefit when used proactively rather than as a last resort.

Putting the Calm Phase Together—A Practical Evening Protocol

The Calm phase tools work best when organized into a consistent evening sequence rather than deployed randomly. Here is a practical protocol that integrates all the elements covered in this chapter into a realistic 90-minute pre-sleep window:

Approximately 90 Minutes Before Bed

- **Take magnesium glycinate** (200 to 400 milligrams elemental magnesium) with water.
- **Take glycine** (3 to 5 grams) dissolved in water, and taurine (500 milligrams to 2 grams) if including it.
- **Take *Mucuna pruriens* if using** (on non-daily strategic occasions, 100 to 300 milligrams of standardized extract).
- **Shift to dimmed, warm lighting** throughout the home. Switch off overhead lights where possible.
- **Put on blue-light-blocking glasses** if screens will be used during this window.

Approximately 30 to 60 Minutes Before Bed

- **Apply essential oils to the legs** (topical lavender blend or magnesium lotion—detailed in Chapter 9).
- **Begin diffusing calming essential oils** in the bedroom if using aromatherapy.
- **Transition to low-arousal activities**—reading, light conversation, gentle stretching, or calm music.
- **Practice two to five minutes of breathwork**—4-7-8 or box breathing before symptoms begin to build.

At Bedtime

- **Ensure the sleeping environment is cool** (65 to 68 degrees Fahrenheit / 18 to 20 degrees Celsius).

- **Eliminate light sources in the room**—blackout curtains or a sleep mask for complete darkness, which optimizes melatonin maintenance through the night.
- **If symptoms are present as you lie down**, deploy the quick-relief tools from Chapter 11 before resorting to getting up—breathwork, topical magnesium lotion on the legs, and position changes are the first line.

Consistency is the mechanism. This protocol does not work dramatically on the first night for most people—it works progressively better over days and weeks as the nervous system begins to associate this sequence of cues with the neurochemical shift toward calm. Like all conditioning effects, it deepens with repetition.

What You Need to Take Away From This Chapter

- **Magnesium glycinate in the evening is the cornerstone of the Calm phase**—it simultaneously reduces glutamate overexcitation through NMDA blockade and enhances GABAergic inhibitory tone, addressing both sides of the excitation-inhibition imbalance in RLS.
- **Magnesium threonate offers superior brain penetration** for those seeking the most neurologically targeted magnesium option, and is worth considering if glycinate produces insufficient relief.
- **Glycine and taurine provide complementary inhibitory neurotransmitter support**, directly enhancing the brain's calming systems through glycine receptor activation, GABA-A agonism, and NMDA modulation.
- ***Mucuna pruriens* is a legitimate short-term dopamine support tool** that can bridge the early months of iron restoration—but must be used strategically, not daily long-term, to avoid the same receptor downregulation that makes pharmaceutical dopamine medications problematic.

- **Morning bright light and evening darkness are the circadian anchors** that determine when melatonin rises and when adenosine can do its calming work undisrupted. Both require deliberate management in the modern light environment.
- **Caffeine after noon directly blunts the adenosine wind-down** during the precise window when RLS symptoms are building. A noon caffeine cutoff is one of the highest-leverage single behavioral changes available.
- **A consistent 90-minute wind-down routine**—combining dimmed lighting, supplement timing, breathwork, and low-arousal activity—creates the neurological conditions for the Calm phase tools to work as effectively as possible.

• • •

In Chapter 9, we turn to essential oils—including the clinical evidence for lavender, the specific mechanisms through which plant compounds interact with the overactivated RLS nervous system, and how to build a practical, effective topical and aromatherapy routine.

CHAPTER NINE

ESSENTIAL OILS FOR RLS RELIEF

Essential oils occupy an interesting position in natural health conversations. For some, they represent the most accessible and instinctively appealing entry point into a more natural approach to wellness. For others, the mention of essential oils immediately raises skepticism—conjuring images of unsubstantiated claims and anecdotal testimonials rather than rigorous science.

Both reactions miss something important. Essential oils are not magic—they are concentrated botanical extracts containing complex mixtures of biologically active compounds that interact with the body's physiological systems through specific, measurable mechanisms. Some of those mechanisms are directly relevant to the neurological picture in RLS. And for one oil in particular—lavender—there is a randomized controlled clinical trial in an RLS-specific population that demonstrates meaningful, measurable benefit.

This chapter approaches essential oils the same way every other intervention in this guide has been approached: from the evidence outward. What does the research actually show? What are the mechanisms? How do these compounds interact with the specific neurochemical systems—sympathetic overactivation, GABA deficiency, nervous system hypersensitivity—that characterize RLS? And then: How do you use them practically, effectively, and safely?

Essential oils in the Calm phase are not a primary intervention in the way that iron restoration is a primary intervention. They are targeted sensory and pharmacological tools that complement the neurochemical support provided by magnesium, glycine, and taurine—and for many people, they provide a degree of immediate, accessible relief that no other tool in the toolkit quite matches in terms of simplicity and speed.

Lavender—The Clinical Evidence

Lavandula angustifolia—true lavender—is the most extensively researched essential oil in the context of sleep, anxiety, and nervous system regulation, and it is the only essential oil with direct clinical evidence for symptom improvement in an RLS-specific population.

The RLS Clinical Trial

A randomized placebo-controlled clinical trial examined the effect of lavender essential oil massage in people undergoing hemodialysis—one of the populations with the highest rates and most severe presentations of RLS. This population was deliberately chosen because the severity and reliability of their RLS symptoms made it possible to detect treatment effects more clearly than in a more heterogeneous outpatient population.

The study compared three groups: a lavender massage group, a reflexology group, and a control massage group. The lavender group received ten drops of diluted lavender essential oil (per foot) massaged into the feet for fifteen minutes on each foot using mild pressure, with specific attention to reflexology points corresponding to the thyroid, parathyroid, pancreas, adrenal glands, and solar plexus. The reflexology group received a standard foot massage with sweet almond oil followed by fifteen minutes of reflexology on the same reflex points. The control group received massage with sweet almond oil only, without targeting specific reflex points.

The protocol was repeated three times per week for eight consecutive weeks. RLS severity was assessed using a validated RLS symptom scale at baseline and throughout the intervention period.

The results were clear and specific: the lavender massage group experienced significant, measurable reductions in RLS severity. The reflexology group and the placebo massage group did not show significant improvement. This finding is important for several reasons. It confirms that the benefit was specific to the lavender oil rather than to massage or reflexology as techniques alone—the control group received equivalent physical contact and the reflexology group received the same structured foot work, and neither produced the same outcome. The active ingredient was the lavender.

> *The key finding of the lavender RLS trial is not simply that lavender helped—it is that it outperformed both massage alone and reflexology alone under controlled conditions. The benefit was attributable to the lavender oil itself, not to touch, attention, or expectation.*

How Lavender Works—The Mechanisms Behind the Benefit

Understanding why lavender works in RLS requires looking at the specific bioactive compounds it contains and how those compounds interact with the neurological systems that drive RLS symptoms. This is not folk medicine—it is polypharmacology applied through a botanical delivery system.

Lavender essential oil is dominated by two primary bioactive compounds: linalool and linalyl acetate (also called linalool acetate), which together typically account for 55 to 80 percent of the oil's composition. Both compounds have well-characterized effects on the central and peripheral nervous system.

Linalool–The GABA Enhancer

Linalool has been shown in multiple studies to enhance GABA-A receptor activity—the same receptor system that glycine and magnesium support through their respective mechanisms.[107] Linalool acts as a positive allosteric modulator of GABA-A receptors,[108] meaning it enhances the receptor's sensitivity to GABA without directly activating it, producing a calming, inhibitory effect on neuronal activity. This mechanism is essentially the same as that of benzodiazepine medications, which work on the same receptor through a related binding site—but linalool does so in a gentler, reversible, and non-habit-forming manner. In other words, it works with your body; it doesn't force it.

Linalool also inhibits voltage-gated calcium channels—a mechanism relevant to both nerve signal propagation and muscle relaxation.[109,110] By reducing calcium entry into neurons, linalool decreases the rate of nerve firing, directly dampening the overactivated sensory and motor signaling that characterizes RLS. In animal studies, linalool consistently produces anxiolytic and sedative effects at doses achievable through aromatherapy and topical application.[111,112]

Sympathetic Nervous System Suppression

Beyond its direct neuroreceptor effects, lavender has documented activity as a suppressor of sympathetic nervous system overactivation. Human studies using heart rate variability analysis—a reliable marker of autonomic nervous system balance—consistently show that lavender inhalation increases parasympathetic (calming) tone and reduces sympathetic (activating) activity.[113] This shift in autonomic balance is measurable within minutes of exposure and is dose-dependent, with longer or more concentrated exposure producing more pronounced effects.

In the RLS context, this is significant because sympathetic overactivation is one of the key drivers of evening symptom escalation. The same nervous system state that characterizes chronic stress—high sympathetic tone, elevated cortisol, suppressed parasympathetic activity—also characterizes the RLS nervous system in the hours before and during symptom onset. Anything that reliably shifts that balance toward parasympathetic dominance directly reduces the neurological backdrop against which RLS symptoms arise.

The Olfactory-Brain Pathway

When lavender is inhaled, volatile compounds reach the olfactory epithelium in the nasal cavity, where olfactory receptor neurons convert them into electrical signals sent directly to the olfactory bulb—one of the most direct routes of chemical communication with the brain available outside of the bloodstream. From the olfactory bulb, signals project to the amygdala (the brain's threat-detection and emotional processing center), the hippocampus, and the limbic system broadly, which governs emotional tone, stress response, and autonomic nervous system regulation.

This olfactory pathway is one of the reasons that aromatherapy can produce nearly instantaneous measurable physiological effects—it is not solely a psychological or placebo mechanism. The compounds in lavender oil reach the limbic system rapidly and directly, activating the parasympathetic nervous system circuitry that produces calming effects before they are even consciously registered as a smell. This is why lavender inhalation studies consistently show heart rate and blood pressure effects occurring within two to five minutes of exposure.

Topical Absorption—The Skin Route

When lavender oil is applied topically to the skin with a carrier oil, its lipophilic (fat-soluble) compounds can permeate the skin barrier and enter the local circulation. Studies measuring lavender compound concentrations in blood following topical massage application confirm that linalool and linalyl acetate are detectable in the bloodstream within 20 minutes of skin application, reaching peak concentrations within 30 to 90 minutes.[114] This systemic absorption means that topical application is not merely a surface-level intervention—the active compounds enter circulation and can reach central nervous system targets.

In the RLS trial, the combination of topical application to the feet and the potential for reflexology-point stimulation may have contributed additional local effects—increased circulation to the lower extremities and direct tissue contact with the skin of the legs and feet, where symptoms are most concentrated. This combined olfactory-and-topical delivery makes lavender foot massage a particularly efficient application method for the RLS relief.

Oral Administration–Lavender From the Inside Out

A growing body of clinical research has examined what happens when lavender oil is taken orally in capsules or softgels—a delivery method that bypasses the olfactory pathway entirely and allows lavender's bioactive compounds to enter systemic circulation through the gastrointestinal tract. The research on this application is substantial, and several of the findings are directly relevant to the RLS nervous system.

The most studied oral protocol involves 80 mg of a standardized lavender oil preparation taken twice daily—160 milligrams total—providing consistent circulating levels of linalool and linalyl acetate throughout the day and evening.[115] Multiple randomized controlled trials have compared this approach to established pharmaceutical anxiolytics, including benzodiazepines and serotonin reuptake inhibitors, for the management of generalized anxiety disorder and related conditions.[116] The results have been consistently meaningful: Oral lavender oil at this dose produces anxiolytic effects comparable in magnitude to those of pharmaceutical medications, with a substantially more favorable side effect profile and no evidence of dependence, tolerance, or withdrawal.

For the person with RLS, the anxiety-reduction effect alone is relevant—anxiety and sympathetic overactivation are among the most reliable amplifiers of evening RLS symptoms, and anything that meaningfully reduces the body's baseline state of arousal reduces the neurological backdrop against which symptoms arise. But the mechanisms that produce these effects are more specifically connected to RLS biology than anxiety reduction alone would suggest.

Oral lavender oil's primary mechanism of action at this dose appears to involve inhibition of voltage-gated calcium channels in neurons—the same channels whose dysregulation contributes to the nerve hyperexcitability and sensory overactivation that characterize RLS.[117] This is mechanistically meaningful: Voltage-gated calcium channel modulation is also the primary mechanism of gabapentin and pregabalin, the alpha-2-delta ligand medications that represent the current first-line pharmaceutical approach to RLS. Oral lavender oil is not intended as a pharmaceutical equivalent, and the magnitude of its effect on these channels differs from those medications—but the directional relevance to neuronal excitability in RLS is real and worth noting.

Research also identifies 5-HT1A serotonin receptor partial agonism as a contributing mechanism—a distinct serotonergic effect that, unlike the broad serotonin reuptake inhibition of SSRIs, does not appear to carry the same risk of worsening RLS.[118] On the contrary, 5-HT1A agonism is associated with autonomic calming and reduced sympathetic tone, supporting the same parasympathetic-dominant state that topical and inhaled lavender promotes through different pathways.

In practical terms, oral lavender oil at 80 milligrams twice daily functions as a systemic nervous system regulator that complements rather than duplicates what topical and inhalation use provides. It reaches tissues that topical application cannot—including deeper nerve structures and the central autonomic circuitry that governs evening arousal—and it maintains a consistent effect throughout the day rather than the time-limited peaks of topical absorption.

How to Use Lavender–Practical Application Methods

There are four primary application methods for lavender in the RLS Calm phase, each with its own strengths and appropriate context. Most people benefit from combining at least two of them in their evening routine.

Topical Application–The Primary Method for RLS

Direct topical application to the legs and feet is the most targeted delivery method for RLS and most closely mirrors what produced results in the clinical trial. Essential oils should always (with very few exceptions) be diluted in a carrier oil before topical use—applying undiluted essential oils directly to skin increases the risk of irritation and can sensitize the skin (make it more prone to reactions) over time, reducing tolerability.

Many people follow a standard dilution for adults of 2 to 5 percent essential oil in carrier oil. For therapeutic use, a 5 percent dilution—which is what was used in the clinical trial—is appropriate and effective. The calculation is straightforward: For a 5 percent dilution in one tablespoon (approximately 15 milliliters) of carrier oil, add 15 drops of lavender essential oil.

The best carrier oils for this application are those that absorb well into the skin, have minimal scent of their own, and provide some skin-nourishing benefit:

- **Sweet almond oil:** The carrier used in the clinical trial. Light, non-greasy, and well tolerated by most skin types. A reliable standard choice. Shelf life 12 to 24 months.
- **Fractionated coconut oil:** Remains liquid at room temperature, absorbs quickly, and is virtually odorless. One

of the most practical and shelf-stable carrier options. Shelf life of 3+ years.

- **Jojoba oil:** Technically a liquid wax ester, closely resembling the skin's own sebum. Excellent for sensitive skin and has a very long shelf life without going rancid. Shelf life 5+ years.
- **Grapeseed oil:** Light, fast-absorbing, and inexpensive. A practical everyday option for those who prefer a less oily feel after application. Shelf life 6 to 18 months.

Application technique: Using the diluted blend, massage the oil into the lower legs and feet using long, moderate-pressure strokes moving upward from the feet toward the knees. Spend at least five minutes on each leg—the clinical trial used fifteen minutes per foot, which is the evidence-based benchmark, though even a briefer application provides meaningful benefit. Focus particular attention on the calves, shins, and the soles of the feet. Warmth from the massage and the friction of application enhances absorption.

Timing: Apply 60 to 90 minutes before bed, during the wind-down window described in Chapter 8. This positions peak plasma levels of lavender compounds to coincide with the typical symptom onset window.

Aromatherapy Diffusion—Ambient Nervous System Support

Diffusing lavender in the bedroom during the wind-down window and through the first hours of sleep provides continuous olfactory input that maintains the parasympathetic shift initiated by topical application. An ultrasonic diffuser that uses water and gentle vibration to disperse essential oil as a fine mist is the safest and most practical option—it does not overheat the oil (which can degrade bioactive compounds and produce irritating byproducts) and runs quietly without disturbing sleep.

A practical starting protocol for diffusion is three to five drops of lavender in a 100-milliliter diffuser, run for 30 to 60 minutes during the wind-down routine and optionally through the first one to two hours of sleep.

People sharing a bedroom with a partner or other household members should consider whether scent preferences and tolerances are compatible. Lavender is among the most broadly tolerated essential oil aromas, but individual variation in preference is significant, and diffusion in a shared sleep environment works best when both parties find the scent pleasant or neutral.

Roller Bottles–Convenient Targeted Application

A pre-blended roller bottle is one of the most practical formats for consistent daily use of lavender— it is easy to apply, easy to carry, and eliminates the need to measure a dilution each time. A 10-milliliter roller bottle at a 5 percent dilution contains approximately 10 drops of essential oil topped up with carrier oil.

The roller format is particularly useful for quick topical application during acute symptom flares—at the first sign of the crawling sensation, rolling directly onto the shins, calves, and soles of the feet provides rapid localized delivery with minimal preparation. It also travels well, making it an accessible tool for the disrupted sleep that often accompanies travel—one of the most challenging environments for people with RLS.

How to Take Lavender Orally–Commercial and DIY Options

There are two practical approaches to oral lavender oil, and both are viable depending on your access to products and preference for convenience.

The simplest option is a commercial enteric-coated lavender oil capsule formulated at the clinically studied level of 80 milligrams of lavender essential oil per capsule. Several such products are available, developed specifically to deliver the lavender oil concentration used in the clinical research. Look for products that clearly state the milligram content of the lavender oil itself—not a lavender extract, standardized concentrate, or herbal preparation—and that specify enteric coating on the label. The enteric coating is important: It prevents the capsule from dissolving prematurely in the gastrointestinal tract for enhanced delivery of the therapeutic compounds and reduced eructation (burp back of volatile compounds). The standard protocol from the clinical research is one 80-milligram capsule taken twice daily—once in the morning and once in the evening, with or without food.

The second option is to make your own capsules at home using size "0" empty gelatin or vegetable capsules, which are widely available and inexpensive. The best type of capsule to use, which mimics enteric coating, are delayed-release (also called acid resistant) capsules. A size "0" capsule holds approximately 0.68 milliliters of liquid when filled. To approximate the 80-milligram clinical dose, add 2 drops of a high-quality lavender essential oil to the capsule body, then fill the remainder of the capsule with a neutral carrier oil—MCT (medium-chain triglycerides from coconut oil), extra-virgin olive oil, or avocado oil all work well. Seal the capsule by fitting the cap over the body and take immediately or store in a sealed container in the refrigerator for up to a week.

A few practical notes on the DIY approach: Standard gelatin capsules will begin to soften if the lavender oil contacts the outer surface, so it is important to fill and cap them promptly. Vegetable cellulose capsules are slightly more resistant to oil contact and are the better choice if you are preparing a small batch in advance rather than making them one at a time. The carrier oil dilutes the lavender and improves oral bioavailability. If you do not use a delayed-release capsule, taking them with a meal rather than on an empty stomach is advisable. If stomach discomfort occurs, a commercial enteric-coated product is the more reliable alternative.

> *Oral lavender oil adds a fourth dimension to the application toolkit—systemic nervous system regulation that works alongside topical, diffusion, and roller bottle methods through entirely different absorption pathways. For people with persistent evening anxiety alongside their RLS, or those whose symptoms have not responded as fully as hoped to topical and aromatherapy approaches alone, oral administration at the clinically studied dose is a logical and well-supported next step.*

Quality and Sourcing—What Matters in Lavender Oil Selection

Essential oil quality is enormously variable, and the lavender category in particular is subject to widespread adulteration—synthetic linalyl acetate or linalool, lavandin oil (a hybrid species with a different chemical profile), and various diluents are commonly used to reduce costs in lower-quality products while maintaining the lavender scent.

For therapeutic use, the following quality indicators matter:

- **Botanical name on the label:** Look for *Lavandula angustifolia* (true lavender) rather than *Lavandula* x *intermedia* (lavandin) or simply "lavender oil." The chemical profiles differ meaningfully—lavandin has higher camphor content and a sharper, less calming scent.
- **GC/MS testing:** Gas chromatography/mass spectrometry is the industry-standard method for verifying essential oil purity and compound composition—but it should not be the only test performed. Reputable companies make GC/MS batch reports available on request or on their websites. A genuine lavender oil should show linalool between 25 and 45 percent and linalyl acetate between 24 and 46 percent, with specific minor components at characteristic ratios, meaning these minor constituents must match nature's precise blueprint to verify the oil's authenticity
- **Country of origin:** The finest therapeutic lavender is produced in the high-altitude regions of Provence in France and Bulgaria. At higher elevations, slower plant maturation produces oils with higher linalool and linalyl acetate concentrations and the smoothest aromatic profiles.
- **Dark glass packaging:** Essential oils oxidize when exposed to light and should be packaged in amber or cobalt blue glass. Avoid products sold in clear glass or plastic bottles.

Additional Supportive Essential Oils

While lavender is the foundation of any essential oil approach to RLS—and the only oil with direct clinical evidence in this population—several other oils have mechanisms and evidence that make them meaningful supporting players. They are best used in combination with lavender, either in blended topical formulas or alongside lavender in a diffuser, rather than as replacements for it.

Roman Chamomile–Relaxation and Anti-Inflammatory Action

Roman chamomile (*Anthemis nobilis* or *Chamaemelum nobile*) is distinct from German chamomile and has a gentler, more apple-like aroma with a particularly strong reputation for calming the nervous system. Its primary bioactive constituents—isobutyl angelate and 2-methylbutyl angelate—have documented sedative and muscle-relaxant properties.[119,120,121] Roman chamomile also contains compounds with mild anti-inflammatory activity,[122] making it a useful complement to lavender in blends targeted at both nervous system calming and the local muscle tension that often accompanies RLS in the legs.

It blends exceptionally well with lavender—the two oils share a broadly calming aromatic character and have complementary, non-overlapping mechanisms of action. In a topical blend, Roman chamomile at one to two percent dilution alongside lavender at three to four percent provides both neural calming and local anti-inflammatory support in a single application.

Marjoram–The Muscle-Soothing Oil

Sweet marjoram (*Origanum majorana*) contains a high concentration of terpinen-4-ol and moderate linalool—compounds with documented muscle relaxant, analgesic, and nervine (nerve-calming) properties.[123,124] In the context of RLS, marjoram is particularly valuable for addressing the muscle tension and secondary discomfort that develops in the calves and legs during symptomatic episodes. It has a warm, herbaceous aroma that most people find grounding rather than alerting.

Applied topically to the calves and shins at one to three percent dilution—or included in a blended formula at that concentration alongside lavender and chamomile—marjoram extends the muscle-relaxant dimension of the topical application that lavender provides primarily through neural mechanisms. It is also a useful addition to the diffuser blend in the bedroom, where its warm, slightly sedating character deepens the overall calming atmosphere.

Frankincense–Nervous System Calm and Anti-Inflammatory Depth

Frankincense (*Boswellia carterii, B. sacra. B. frereana, B. papyrifera*) is one of the most pharmacologically complex essential oils available, with over 300 identified chemical constituents. Its primary therapeutic compounds—alpha-pinene and limonene—have demonstrated anti-inflammatory, neuroprotective, and anxiolytic properties in research settings.[125]

For RLS, frankincense is most relevant as a nervous system regulator with a grounding, centering quality that complements the lighter floral character of lavender. Research on the diterpene found in frankincense, incensole acetate, discovered that inhalation reduces anxiety and depressive-like symptoms, and *in vitro* studies suggest it is a potent modulator of ion channels relevant to nerve signaling—a mechanism similar in direction to lavender's calcium channel effects, though through different specific channels.[126] In blended formulas, frankincense adds aromatic depth and extends the anti-inflammatory benefit of the overall blend.

Rosemary–Circulation and Local Inflammation

Rosemary (*Salvia rosmarinus* or *Rosmarinus officinalis*; specifically the camphor chemotype or the 1,8-cineole chemotype) improves local circulation when applied topically—a benefit that is relevant to the leg discomfort component of RLS, where reduced circulation in the legs during periods of inactivity can contribute to the uncomfortable sensations driving the urge to move.[127]

An important note: Rosemary is more stimulating than the other oils in this section and should be used specifically in the topical leg massage blend rather than in the diffuser blend for the bedroom—its invigorating quality makes it counterproductive as an ambient aromatherapy choice in the sleep environment. In topical application to the legs, its circulatory benefit is a useful addition to the calming and muscle-relaxant effects of the other oils.

Copaiba–Anti-Inflammatory and CNS Calming

Copaiba (*Copaifera* spp.) is an oil derived from the resin of South American copaiba trees and is extraordinarily rich in beta-caryophyllene—a sesquiterpene compound that is one of the few plant-derived substances known to directly activate the CB2 cannabinoid receptor. CB2 receptors are found throughout the peripheral nervous system and immune system, and their activation produces anti-inflammatory and analgesic effects without the psychoactive properties associated with CB1 activation.[128]

Additionally, a randomized controlled human trial found that inhaling copaiba essential oil from an atomizing diffuser reduces anxiety.[129] The diffuser was set to intermittent while participants inhaled the aroma. They then participated in a mental load task involving mental arithmetic. Heart rate, salivary cortisol, and self-reported anxiety all decreased in the copaiba group compared to the control (jojoba oil only). In addition, a remarkable reduction in beta wave activity was observed in the left midfrontal region (F3) of the brain when participants inhaled copaiba oil. Since RLS is a central nervous system disorder, the reduction at F3—an area of the brain involved in executive function, motor planning, and the regulation of emotional and physical restlessness—represents the objective "brain signature" of the sedative and muscle-relaxant effects needed to counteract the hyperarousal of RLS.

This CB2-mediated anti-inflammatory activity and its nervous system effects make copaiba a meaningful complement to lavender in RLS blends—it adds an additional layer of nervous system calming and peripheral anti-inflammatory support through a completely different receptor pathway. Beta-caryophyllene is also found in black pepper, cloves, and hops essential oils, but copaiba has by far the highest concentration of any common essential oil. In a topical blend at one to two percent, it contributes to both local anti-inflammatory effect in the legs and broader calming through its systemic absorption.

Building Practical Blends—Formulas for Everyday Use

The following blends are evidence-informed and designed to be practical and easy to prepare at home with commonly available ingredients. All are formulated at a 5 percent total essential oil dilution in a carrier oil base. Dilutions are calculated for a 10-milliliter roller bottle, which provides approximately two to three weeks of daily application.

The Core RLS Blend–Topical Leg Application

This blend most closely mirrors the clinical trial protocol while incorporating the complementary mechanisms of the supporting oils. It is the starting point recommended for most people.

- **Lavender:** 6 drops
- **Roman chamomile:** 2 drops
- **Marjoram:** 2 drops
- **Carrier oil (fractionated coconut or sweet almond):** fill roller bottle to 10 milliliters

Apply to the calves, shins, and soles of the feet 60 to 90 minutes before bed. Massage in using upward strokes from ankle to knee. For acute flares, apply at the first sign of symptoms.

The Deep Calm Blend–Enhanced Nervous System Support

For people with more significant nervous system overactivation—severe or highly unpredictable evening symptoms, high stress, or a more reactive baseline—this blend adds the deeper anti-inflammatory and calming layers of frankincense and copaiba.

- **Lavender:** 5 drops
- **Frankincense:** 2 drops
- **Copaiba:** 2 drops
- **Roman chamomile:** 1 drop
- **Carrier oil:** fill roller bottle to 10 milliliters

Use topically on the legs as with the Core RLS Blend. Frankincense and copaiba can also be applied to the back of the neck, wrists, and chest to extend the overall calming effect.

The Bedroom Diffuser Blend—Ambient Sleep Support

This diffuser blend is designed for the sleep environment—calming without being sedating to the point of morning grogginess, with a combined aromatic character that supports the parasympathetic wind-down without the stimulating elements that make rosemary inappropriate for this context.

- **Lavender:** 2 drops
- **Roman chamomile:** 2 drops
- **Copaiba:** 2 drops
- **Frankincense:** 1 drop

Add to a 100-milliliter ultrasonic diffuser with water. Run for 30 to 60 minutes during the wind-down routine, using the diffuser's intermittent cycle setting if available. Can be left running overnight while sleeping, if desired.

The Circulation and Comfort Blend—Topical Leg Rub for Acute Symptoms

This blend is specifically designed for acute symptom relief—when the crawling sensations and urge to move are actively present and something more targeted than the standard bedtime routine is needed. The addition of rosemary for its circulatory benefit and the slightly higher lavender concentration distinguish it from the general maintenance blends.

- **Lavender:** 5 drops
- **Marjoram:** 3 drops
- **Rosemary (1,8-cineole chemotype):** 2 drops
- **Carrier oil:** fill roller bottle to 10 milliliters

Apply directly to the affected legs with firm upward strokes when symptoms are active. The circulatory stimulation from rosemary combined with the neural calming from lavender and marjoram addresses both the vascular and neurological components of acute symptom discomfort. Because this blend contains rosemary, it is for topical leg application only—not for diffusion in the sleep environment.

> *Having two formats ready—a maintenance roller for the nightly wind-down routine and an acute relief roller for when symptoms flare unexpectedly—means you are never without a fast-acting tool. The two-minute act of rolling and massaging a blend into your legs can provide meaningful relief within 15 to 20 minutes through both topical absorption and the olfactory calming response.*

Safety Guidelines—Using Essential Oils Responsibly

Essential oils are potent botanical concentrates, and responsible use requires attention to a few reasonable safety principles. These are not intended to create anxiety around their use—properly diluted essential oils are safe for the vast majority of adults—but to prevent the small number of issues that arise from misuse.

- **Always dilute before topical application**—undiluted essential oils should rarely be applied directly to skin for therapeutic use. The 5 percent dilution used in the clinical trial is appropriate for targeted therapeutic application. For general daily maintenance use, a 2 to 3 percent dilution may be more appropriate for prolonged use.
- **Patch test before full application**—apply a small amount of the diluted blend to the inner forearm and wait 24 hours before using it on larger skin areas. Sensitivity reactions, while uncommon with properly diluted oils, are more likely in people with a compromised immune system—

autoimmunity, autoinflammation, seasonal allergies, food allergies, eczema, psoriasis, or known plant allergies.

- **Pregnancy considerations**—some essential oils are contraindicated in pregnancy. Lavender, frankincense, copaiba, and Roman chamomile are generally considered safe at appropriate dilutions during pregnancy, but rosemary should be avoided. Anyone who is pregnant should review specific oil safety with a knowledgeable healthcare provider before use.
- **Medication interactions**—at normal topical and aromatherapy doses, essential oils are unlikely to produce clinically significant drug interactions. However, people should consult Appendix G of *Medicinal Essential Oils* for potential drug interactions and then discuss the information with their prescribing clinician before beginning a regular therapeutic essential oil routine.
- **Store properly**—in a cool, dark location away from heat and direct light. Pre-blended roller bottles should be used within six to twelve months for optimal potency.

What You Need to Take Away From This Chapter

- **Lavender essential oil has clinical evidence for reducing RLS severity** in a hemodialysis population—a finding that reflects specific pharmacological mechanisms, not placebo or touch effects.
- **Linalool and linalyl acetate—lavender's primary bioactive compounds—act through GABA-A receptor potentiation, calcium channel inhibition, and sympathetic nervous system suppression**: three mechanisms directly relevant to the neurochemical picture of RLS.
- **Topical application to the legs and feet is the primary delivery method for RLS**, at a 5 percent dilution in a carrier oil, massaged for at least five minutes per leg during the wind-down window.

- **Diffusion in the bedroom during the wind-down routine** provides complementary olfactory-pathway calming that deepens the parasympathetic shift initiated by topical application.
- **Oral use of lavender oil** reaches tissues that topical application cannot and sustains the effects throughout the day.
- **Roman chamomile, marjoram, frankincense, rosemary, and copaiba** each offer complementary mechanisms—muscle relaxation, additional GABA support, CB2 anti-inflammatory activity, and improved circulation—that enhance the effectiveness of lavender in blended formulas.
- **Quality matters**: Source lavender specifically, look for GC/MS testing documentation, and choose products from reputable suppliers with transparent sourcing to ensure that therapeutic compound concentrations are present in the oil being used.

• • •

In Chapter 10, all three phases of the framework come together into a complete, practical daily protocol—a morning-to-evening routine that makes the full strategy accessible, sustainable, and livable.

CHAPTER TEN

THE PRACTICAL DAILY PROTOCOL

Five chapters of practical strategy. A clear framework. Specific foods, supplements, essential oils, timing protocols, and behavioral guidance—all grounded in the biology of what is actually happening in the RLS brain. The science is there. The tools are there. What remains is the question every serious reader arrives at eventually: How does all of this actually fit into a day?

This chapter answers that question. It takes everything from the Restore, Deliver, and Calm phases and organizes it into a realistic daily structure—morning, midday, and evening—that is practical for people with real lives, variable schedules, and something other than RLS management to think about during the day.

A few design principles before the protocol itself. First, this is a framework, not a rigid prescription. The goal is not perfect adherence to every element every day—it is a consistent direction of daily behavior that compounds over time. Missing a supplement, skipping a meal element, or cutting the evening routine short on a difficult night does not undo progress. Consistency over weeks matters far more than perfection on any given day.

Second, the protocol is designed to be built gradually. For most people, implementing everything at once creates an overwhelming cognitive load that leads to abandonment within two weeks. A better approach is to add one new practice every few days, allowing each to become automatic before the next is introduced. By the end of the first month, what initially felt like a lot of moving pieces will have settled into a routine that requires relatively little conscious effort to maintain.

Third, the evening window is disproportionately important. Morning and midday practices support the strategy, but the evening is where RLS wins or loses on any given night. The evening protocol receives the most detail in this chapter for precisely that reason.

Morning—Setting the Foundation for the Day

The morning window serves two functions in the RLS daily protocol. The first is biological: Morning practices set the circadian anchor that will determine the quality of the evening wind-down twelve to sixteen hours later. The second is nutritional: The morning is the optimal window for iron supplementation, and a well-structured breakfast begins the dietary iron and anti-inflammatory work that the day builds upon.

Neither function requires dramatic changes to a morning routine. The practices below can be integrated into even a compressed morning without adding significant time.

Light Exposure—Within the First Hour of Waking

Getting outside for natural light—or sitting near a window or light therapy lamp—within the first 60 minutes of waking is the single most powerful circadian anchor available. It does not need to be long:

Ten to twenty minutes of exposure to natural or broad-spectrum bright light is sufficient to trigger the hormonal cascade that sets the biological clock for the day. On clear days, eating breakfast near a window or doing a brief outdoor walk accomplishes this without any additional time commitment.

In winter months or in climates with limited natural light, a 10,000-lux broad-spectrum light therapy lamp positioned at eye level for 20 minutes during breakfast produces equivalent benefits. This is also particularly useful for people who need to be up well before dawn—the artificial bright light substitutes for the sunrise signal the circadian system needs.

Iron Supplementation—Before Breakfast on Alternate Days

On alternate mornings, take iron supplementation before breakfast—on an empty stomach, with 100 to 250 milligrams of vitamin C, and well before coffee or tea. This timing exploits the morning window when hepcidin is naturally at its lowest, maximizing absorption from each dose. Set a consistent schedule—Monday, Wednesday, Friday, Sunday, for example—so that alternate-day dosing becomes automatic rather than something that requires daily decision-making.

On iron supplement days, delay coffee or tea by at least 60 minutes after taking the supplement. This is the single most commonly violated timing rule in iron supplementation, and it meaningfully undermines absorption when ignored. If delaying coffee feels impossible in the early adjustment period, set the coffee maker on a timer to begin brewing 60 minutes after you plan to take your supplement—removing the decision entirely.

Oral Lavender—Morning Dose If Using

For those incorporating oral lavender oil as discussed in Chapter 9, the morning dose is taken at breakfast—with food to improve tolerability if using a DIY capsule without enteric coating. The morning dose maintains daytime circulating levels of linalool and linalyl acetate that support sustained calcium channel modulation and autonomic tone throughout the day, reducing the sympathetic baseline that RLS symptoms build upon by evening.

A Protein-Rich Breakfast—Iron, Cofactors, and Sustained Energy

Breakfast is not a minor nutritional event in the RLS protocol—it is an opportunity to front-load the heme iron, cofactor nutrients, and protein that the day's biology depends on. A breakfast built around animal protein provides heme iron, B vitamins, zinc, and complete amino acids in a single meal. Eggs with smoked salmon or sardines, a beef-based breakfast, or full-fat yogurt with seeds and berries are all practical and nutrient-dense options that require minimal preparation.

If liver is included in the diet—ideally one to two times per week—breakfast or lunch is typically the most practical meal for it. A small amount of beef liver cooked with eggs and onions, or a liver-containing sausage or pâté on whole-grain toast, provides a concentrated dose of iron, copper, and retinol that dietary supplementation alone struggles to replicate.

Avoid starting the day with a purely carbohydrate-based breakfast—cereal, toast, pastries, or sweetened yogurt—not because carbohydrates are inherently problematic, but because these choices provide minimal iron, none of the cofactor nutrition the strategy depends on, and contribute to the blood sugar instability and inflammatory signaling that the Deliver phase is working to reduce.

Morning Supplements

The morning supplement window accommodates the anti-inflammatory and Deliver phase nutrients that are best taken with food for absorption and tolerability. A practical morning supplement stack for most people implementing this protocol includes:

- **Omega-3 (fish oil or algae oil):** 1,000 to 2,000 milligrams EPA plus DHA, taken with breakfast. Fat-soluble and best absorbed with a meal containing dietary fat.
- **Vitamin D3 with K2:** taken with the fattiest meal of the day—for most people this is breakfast or lunch. Vitamin D is fat-soluble, and absorption drops significantly when taken without dietary fat.
- **Curcumin (if included):** taken with a fat-containing meal, separated from iron by at least two hours. Morning with breakfast works well for most people.
- **Oral lavender capsule (if using):** first dose taken with breakfast as noted above.
- **Probiotic (if included):** taken with breakfast—with a meal is most important. Store in the refrigerator to maintain maximum potency.

> *Morning light within 60 minutes of waking and morning iron before breakfast on alternate days are the two highest-leverage morning practices in the entire protocol. Everything else in the morning routine builds on the foundation those two create.*

Midday—Sustaining the Nutritional and Inflammatory Strategy

The midday window has a simpler role than morning or evening: It is primarily about sustaining the dietary and anti-inflammatory work without actively undermining the evening Calm phase that is still hours away. A few key practices keep the strategy moving forward through the middle of the day.

A Nutrient-Dense Lunch—Iron, Color, and Quality Fat

Lunch is the second major dietary iron opportunity of the day and the ideal window for including fatty fish if it is not already part of breakfast. A practical midday framework: a protein source providing heme iron or omega-3s—red meat, salmon, sardines, poultry dark meat, or shellfish—alongside a variety of colorful vegetables dressed with olive oil, and a whole-food carbohydrate if needed for energy. This combination provides anti-inflammatory polyphenols, further iron contribution, gut-supporting fiber, and the sustained energy that prevents the blood sugar dips that increase cortisol and worsen afternoon stress.

Including a fermented food at lunch—a tablespoon of sauerkraut alongside the meal, a side of plain yogurt, or miso in a soup—adds the daily microbiome support that the Deliver phase depends on without requiring any additional thought or effort beyond keeping these items stocked.

Movement—The Midday Circulation Reset

Moderate movement during the day is one of the most consistently beneficial non-supplement interventions for RLS. Regular exercise—even modest amounts—supports dopaminergic function, reduces

CRP and inflammatory markers over time, improves sleep architecture, and provides direct short-term relief from RLS symptoms through mechanisms that include increased dopamine availability and improved peripheral circulation.[130,131,132]

The practical guidance is deliberately moderate: twenty to forty minutes of activity at a conversational pace, three to five times per week. Walking, cycling, swimming, strength training, mobility, or any low-to-moderate-impact activity qualifies. High-intensity or excessively long training sessions can worsen RLS through the iron-depletion and cortisol-elevation mechanisms discussed in Chapter 4, making moderate exercise a better fit than performance-oriented training for people in active RLS recovery.

Timing matters for RLS specifically. Exercise earlier in the day—morning or early afternoon—provides all the dopaminergic and cardiovascular benefits without the body temperature elevation and sympathetic nervous system activation that late-day vigorous exercise can introduce in the evening hours. As a general rule, completing any meaningful physical activity at least four to five hours before bed minimizes its potential interference with the evening calming protocol.

Caffeine Cutoff—No Later Than Noon

Midday marks the caffeine cutoff. As established in Chapter 8, the five-to-seven-hour half-life of caffeine means that anything consumed after noon is still meaningfully active in the adenosine system during the peak RLS risk window of 9 to 11 p.m. This is not a suggestion—for people with moderate to severe evening symptoms, it is one of the most impactful single behavioral changes available, and it costs nothing except the habit of an afternoon coffee or tea.

For people who rely on an afternoon caffeine boost to maintain energy through the workday, this is often a sign that sleep quality is insufficiently restorative—which is a consequence of RLS itself, creating a dependency cycle where poor RLS sleep drives afternoon caffeine need, which worsens RLS sleep. Breaking this cycle typically requires a short-term period of afternoon fatigue while sleep quality gradually improves, after which the afternoon energy dip resolves on its own.

Midday Stress Management–Brief and Consistent

For people with high chronic stress loads, a brief midday decompression practice makes a meaningful contribution to the overall inflammatory reduction that the Deliver phase requires. This does not need to be elaborate: five to ten minutes of slow diaphragmatic breathing, a short walk outdoors, or simply stepping away from work demands during lunch without screens represents a reliable cortisol and inflammation management practice that compounds over weeks. The goal is not stress elimination—it is reducing the degree to which midday stress accumulates and carries forward into the evening neurological environment.

The Afternoon Transition–Preparing the Evening Environment

The two to three hours before the evening wind-down routine is a transition zone—the period when daily demands are winding down but the active Calm phase protocol has not yet begun. A few specific practices during this window meaningfully extend the effectiveness of the evening routine by reducing the physiological arousal state that the evening tools are working to calm.

A Light, Early Dinner—Timing and Composition

A relatively early dinner—ideally completed two to three hours before bed—serves several functions simultaneously. It allows the digestive process to complete before sleep onset, preventing the metabolic activation of active digestion from interfering with the neurological calming process of the wind-down. It also avoids late-evening blood sugar fluctuations, which can spike cortisol and worsen the sympathetic activation that evening RLS builds on.

Dinner composition follows the same anti-inflammatory, protein-anchored approach as the rest of the day, with one practical addition: including foods that contribute to the calming neurotransmitter environment of the evening. Tryptophan-rich foods—turkey, chicken, eggs, dairy, seeds—provide a dietary precursor to serotonin and subsequently melatonin, supporting natural sleep onset. Magnesium-rich foods—dark leafy greens, seeds, nuts, dark chocolate (keep it to about one ounce to avoid too much caffeine)—add to the tissue magnesium that the supplement is building. Neither of these requires a specific "sleep-supporting dinner" concept—they are simply naturally present in a diverse, whole-food evening meal.

Alcohol warrants specific mention here. A glass of wine or beer in the evening is a common relaxation choice that, for people with RLS, typically makes the night worse despite initially feeling calming. Alcohol is a GABA agonist and initially produces sedation—but as it metabolizes, it produces a rebound excitatory effect in the second half of the night that fragments sleep architecture, reduces REM and slow-wave sleep, elevates inflammatory markers, and worsens the neurological conditions that drive RLS.[133] It also directly depletes magnesium.[134] For people in active RLS recovery, removing evening alcohol—at least as a consistent experiment—is worth the trial.

Reducing Screen and Cognitive Demand—The Pre-Wind-Down Wind-Down

The most common obstacle to an effective evening wind-down is not a lack of time—it is arriving at the wind-down window already in a state of high cognitive and emotional arousal from evening news consumption, work emails, emotionally engaging social media, or stressful conversations. The brain does not transition from high arousal to calm rest in the space of a supplement dose and dimmed lights. It needs a gradual ramp-down.

In the two hours before the active wind-down routine begins, reducing the intensity of incoming cognitive and emotional stimulation allows the nervous system to begin its own natural descent before any deliberate calming tools are introduced. This does not require a media blackout—it means replacing high-stimulation content with lower-stimulation alternatives: a novel instead of the news, a gentle podcast instead of a debate, a phone call with a friend instead of scrolling social media.

Evening—The Critical Window

The evening is where the strategy is won or lost each night. Every practice from Chapters 8 and 9 converges here—supplements, essential oils, light management, breathwork, and the environmental conditions that allow the nervous system to genuinely downregulate. The protocol below represents the full implementation of the Calm phase across a 90-minute pre-sleep window.

Not every element will be implemented from day one—and that is the correct approach. Start with the two or three practices that feel most accessible, establish those as habit, then add the next layer. The full protocol as described below is the destination to build toward over three to four weeks, not a requirement from the first night.

90 Minutes Before Bed—The Supplement and Environment Shift

This is the most important single transition point in the entire daily protocol. Everything that follows becomes easier and more effective when this window is used well.

- **Take magnesium glycinate**—200 to 400 milligrams of elemental magnesium. This is the cornerstone evening supplement. Taking it 90 minutes before bed positions absorption and peak tissue levels to coincide with the symptom onset window.
- **Take glycine and taurine**—3 to 5 grams of glycine powder dissolved in water, and 500 milligrams to 2 grams of taurine. These can be combined in the same glass. The mild sweetness of glycine makes this a pleasant, easy-to-take evening drink.
- **Take oral lavender capsule if using**—the evening dose, with or without a small amount of food as appropriate for the preparation used.
- **Take *Mucuna pruriens* on strategic occasions**—not every night, but on nights when symptoms are expected to be more severe, travel disrupts the usual routine, or during the early weeks before iron restoration has produced meaningful improvement.
- **Shift to warm, dimmed lighting**—turn off overhead lights and switch to lamps, candles, or other low-level warm

light sources throughout the home. This is the environmental signal that initiates the melatonin onset process.

- **Put on blue-light-blocking glasses** if screens will be used during this window. Enable night mode or warm color shift on all devices.

60 Minutes Before Bed—The Oils and Wind-Down Practice

- **Begin diffusing lavender and supportive essential oils** in the bedroom—the bedroom diffuser blend from Chapter 9, or plain lavender at five to seven drops in a 100-milliliter diffuser.
- **Apply the essential oil blend to the legs**—using the Core RLS Blend or Deep Calm Blend from Chapter 9, rolled or massaged into the calves, shins, and soles of the feet. Spend at least five minutes per leg using upward strokes. This is not incidental—this is the topical delivery method that produced the clinical trial results.
- **Transition to low-arousal activity**—reading a physical book, light stretching, calm music, or quiet conversation. Anything that does not involve news, work, or emotionally engaging content.
- **Practice breathwork—proactively, before symptoms build**. Two to five minutes of 4-7-8 breathing or box breathing done before the RLS crawling sensation arrives is significantly more effective than deploying it after symptoms have already peaked. This is the nervous system's emergency brake—use it before you need it urgently.
- **Apply topical magnesium lotion to the legs** if it is part of the routine—after the essential oil application and before bed, as a complementary topical layer.

At Bedtime—The Final Environmental Setup

- **Cool the sleeping environment** to 65 to 68 degrees Fahrenheit (18 to 20 degrees Celsius). If this is not possible through thermostat control, a fan directed at the bed, cooling sheets, or a hot-then-cool shower before bed (which accelerates core temperature drop) all provide meaningful support.
- **Eliminate light from the sleeping environment**—blackout curtains, tape over indicator lights, a sleep mask if needed. Even small amounts of light during sleep suppress melatonin and fragment sleep architecture.
- **Go to bed at the same time each night**—within a 30-minute consistency window, including weekends. This regularity is what builds the reliable circadian melatonin rhythm that makes sleep onset progressively easier over time.
- **If symptoms are present as you lie down**, deploy the quick-relief toolkit from Chapter 11 before getting up—the acute-relief roller blend, topical magnesium, a brief repositioning or stretch, and another round of slow breathing are all first-line responses that often interrupt the symptom cycle without requiring full movement.

> *The evening protocol is a sequence, not a list of individual items. Each element creates the conditions for the next to work more effectively. Dimmed lights prepare the melatonin environment. Supplements absorbed 90 minutes out are at peak effect when symptoms typically begin. Oil applied to the legs is reaching peak plasma levels as you lie down. Breathwork done before symptoms arrive prevents the escalation that makes symptoms feel unmanageable. The sequence is the mechanism.*

Weekly and Periodic Practices—What Does Not Need to Be Daily

Not everything in the strategy needs to happen every day. Several important practices are most effective and most sustainable when built into a weekly rhythm rather than a daily obligation.

- **Liver, once to twice per week:** This frequency provides the most impactful combined dose of heme iron, copper, retinol, and B vitamins available through food, without creating the vitamin A accumulation risk that could theoretically arise from daily consumption of very large amounts.
- **Fatty fish, two to three times per week:** Salmon, sardines, mackerel, or herring at this frequency provides the EPA and DHA foundation that renders daily fish oil supplementation optional rather than essential.
- **Iron testing, every eight to twelve weeks:** Ferritin, transferrin saturation, and CRP checked together provide the objective scorecard of Restore and Deliver phase progress. Schedule tests proactively rather than waiting until symptoms worsen to check in with the numbers.
- **Prepare essential oil blends in batches:** A 10-milliliter roller bottle lasts two to three weeks with daily use. Setting aside five minutes every few weeks to prepare the next batch ensures the tool is always ready when needed.
- **A weekly protocol review:** Spending five minutes on Sunday noting what worked, what was missed, and what to adjust in the coming week creates the habit of deliberate course-correction without requiring daily self-monitoring that becomes burdensome.

Adapting the Protocol to Real Life

A daily protocol designed in ideal conditions needs to be flexible enough to survive the conditions of an actual life—travel, work events, family demands, illness, and the thousand ordinary disruptions that mean any given day may not look like the framework above. A few principles for maintaining the strategy through real-world variation:

When Traveling

Travel is one of the most challenging environments for RLS—prolonged sitting, disrupted sleep timing, jet lag, different food environments, and limited access to usual routines combine to create conditions that reliably worsen symptoms. A compact travel kit that preserves the most essential Calm phase tools makes an enormous practical difference: an acute-relief roller bottle, magnesium glycinate capsules, glycine powder in a small container, and oral lavender capsules if using. These fit into a personal bag and maintain the most impactful elements of the evening protocol regardless of accommodation or schedule.

On flights, apply the acute-relief roller blend to the legs before boarding and during the flight at the first sign of symptom onset. Take magnesium and glycine with water during the flight rather than waiting for the hotel. Walk the aisle briefly every 60 to 90 minutes during long flights—movement is one of the most reliable short-term symptom interrupters available, and brief walks are specifically permitted precisely because sitting still for hours is one of the most powerful RLS triggers.

On High-Demand or High-Stress Days

On days when chronic stress is unusually high—a difficult work period, family crisis, or significant life event—RLS symptoms are often more severe in the evening, reflecting the cortisol and sympathetic overactivation that high-demand days produce. On these nights, the protocol matters more, not less. A concrete response to high-stress days is to double down on the most impactful Calm phase practices rather than abandoning them: extra attention to the full evening routine, proactive breathwork earlier in the evening, and the generous application of essential oil blends before symptoms build.

When a Good Night Becomes Complacency

One of the most common patterns in RLS recovery is this: Several nights of meaningful improvement lead to the conclusion that the protocol can be relaxed—supplements skipped, evening routine abbreviated, caffeine cutoff extended. The following nights are often the worst in weeks. This is not a coincidence. The biological systems underlying RLS do not retain their improved state without ongoing support—particularly during the months before iron restoration is complete and the nervous system can self-regulate more reliably.

Good nights are confirmation that the strategy is working—not permission to stop executing it. The correct response to improvement is gratitude and continuation, not relaxation and drift.

Tracking Progress—Making the Invisible Visible

RLS recovery is gradual enough that it can be difficult to perceive without a systematic way of tracking it. A week that feels discouraging often looks dramatically better when compared to the baseline recorded six weeks earlier. Tracking does not need to be elaborate—a simple nightly log of symptom severity on a scale of zero to ten, sleep quality rating, and any notable protocol deviations takes less than two minutes and creates a data record that makes progress visible and helps identify patterns.

The most useful things to track alongside symptom severity are ferritin at each testing interval, protocol adherence for key practices (iron supplement day yes or no, evening routine completed yes or partial), and any notable lifestyle factors—travel, unusual stress, exercise type and intensity, dietary deviations. Over weeks, patterns emerge: which practices correlate most strongly with better nights, which lapses produce the sharpest symptom rebounds, how ferritin changes relate to subjective symptom trends.

This kind of self-monitoring is not about creating anxiety or perfectionism—it is about building an evidence base for your own particular biology so that adjustments to the protocol are guided by data rather than intuition alone.

What You Need to Take Away From This Chapter

- **The morning window sets the biological foundation**—light exposure anchors the circadian clock and alternate-day iron supplementation before breakfast exploits the natural low-hepcidin morning window.
- **Midday sustains and protects**—a nutrient-dense lunch, the caffeine cutoff at noon, moderate exercise earlier in the day, and brief stress management practices keep the strategy moving without requiring significant disruption to daytime routines.
- **The evening protocol is where the night is decided**—the 90-minute wind-down window, properly sequenced, positions every Calm phase tool at peak effectiveness during the highest-risk symptom window.
- **The sequence is the mechanism**—dimmed lights, supplements, oils, breathwork, and temperature control are not independent choices. They build on each other in a specific order that the nervous system learns to associate with safety and rest.

- **Build gradually, not all at once**—implementing one to two new practices every few days produces more durable habit formation than attempting the full protocol from day one.
- **Good nights require continued execution, not relaxation**—the protocol that produced improvement is the protocol that sustains it, particularly during the months before iron restoration is complete.

• • •

In Chapter 11, we turn to the quick-relief toolkit—what to do in the moment when symptoms hit acutely, with fast-acting strategies organized for immediate use.

CHAPTER ELEVEN

THE QUICK RELIEF TOOLKIT—WHEN SYMPTOMS HIT

It is 10:30 at night. You have done everything right today. Iron supplement taken in the morning. Good dinner. Evening supplements at 9:00. Legs oiled. Lights dimmed. You lay down—and within minutes, the crawling starts.

This is the reality of RLS recovery. The protocol reduces the frequency and severity of symptom episodes over time, but it does not produce an impenetrable shield around every night—especially in the early months before iron restoration has produced meaningful neurochemical improvement. Symptoms will still arrive on some nights. The question is not how to prevent every single episode but how to interrupt it quickly, minimize its duration, and return to rest rather than lying awake for hours escalating the very sympathetic overactivation that makes symptoms worse.

This chapter is a practical, immediately deployable toolkit for those moments. Each tool has a specific mechanism, a specific technique, and a specific place in the response sequence. Together they form a layered response system—starting with the least disruptive interventions and escalating to more active strategies only if earlier ones are insufficient.

One framing note: The goal of the quick-relief toolkit is interruption and return to rest—not perfect, immediate symptom elimination. Most of these tools work by disrupting the sensory-escalation cycle and giving the nervous system a window to settle. Applying them with that expectation produces better results and less frustration than expecting symptoms to vanish in sixty seconds.

The Response Hierarchy—A Layered Approach

Not all symptom episodes are equal. A mild crawling sensation that started 10 minutes ago responds to different tools than a severe, full-leg episode that has been building for an hour. And some tools—particularly those involving getting out of bed and moving—provide reliable relief but at the cost of further alerting the nervous system, making sleep reinstatement harder. The following sequence moves from least disruptive to most disruptive, providing the best chance of relief while preserving the conditions for returning to sleep.

- **Tier 1—In-bed interventions:** breathwork, topical oil application, magnesium lotion, positional changes. Use these first. They interrupt the symptom cycle without requiring full waking or movement.
- **Tier 2—Minimal movement:** targeted stretching performed at the bedside, brief pressure application, massage techniques. These involve some movement but can be completed in two to three minutes without leaving the sleep environment.
- **Tier 3—Active relief:** walking, temperature therapy, full-body movement. These are the most reliable symptom interrupters but involve leaving the bedroom and more fully

alerting the nervous system. Use when Tier 1 and 2 have been genuinely attempted without adequate relief.

> *The worst response to early-stage symptoms is anxious waiting—lying still, tensing against the sensations, and watching them grow. Anxiety about the symptoms amplifies the sympathetic activation that drives them. Responding actively and calmly, with a specific tool, interrupts this amplification cycle and gives the nervous system a more productive direction.*

Tier 1–In-Bed Interventions

Breathwork–The First Response

When symptoms first begin, before reaching for anything else, deploy slow diaphragmatic breathing. This is the first tool for a reason: It is immediately available, requires nothing but your own breath, and directly activates the vagal brake that shifts the nervous system away from the sympathetic overactivation driving the symptom escalation.

The mechanism matters here. The sympathetic nervous system generates the sensory amplification that makes RLS symptoms feel so urgent and unignorable. Slow exhalation—specifically, making the exhale longer than the inhale—stimulates the vagus nerve and activates parasympathetic dominance within two to three breathing cycles. This does not eliminate the RLS signal, but it measurably reduces the nervous system's sensitivity to it, lowering the threshold at which the sensations become unbearable.

The acute response protocol: Inhale slowly through the nose for a count of four, hold for two, exhale through the mouth for a count of six to eight. Repeat this six to eight times before assessing whether symptoms are beginning to settle. The extended exhale is the active mechanism—the longer the exhale relative to the inhale, the stronger the vagal activation. Do not rush through the cycles. Slow and deliberate is more effective than fast and mechanical.

If this level of breath control feels difficult while symptoms are active, a simpler version—breathe out for twice as long as you breathe in, at whatever count feels natural—achieves the same effect. The ratio is what matters more than the specific numbers.

Topical Essential Oil Application—In Bed, Immediately

Having the acute-relief roller blend from Chapter 9 on the bedside table means it is available within arm's reach when symptoms begin—no need to get up, turn on lights, or prepare anything. Roll it directly onto the calves and shins while lying in bed, using firm strokes from ankle upward to knee, and repeat on both legs even if only one is symptomatic. The olfactory response begins within two to three minutes of smelling the blend as you apply it, and the topical compounds begin absorbing immediately.

This intervention pairs powerfully with breathwork—applying the oil while continuing slow exhale-extended breathing creates a simultaneous sensory-calming and neurological-calming effect. The smell of lavender while practicing slow breathing reinforces the association between the scent and the calming state that the evening routine has been building, making the olfactory response progressively faster and stronger with consistent use over weeks.

A second application five to ten minutes after the first, if symptoms are still present, is entirely appropriate. There is no meaningful risk of overusing a properly diluted topical essential oil blend. Repeat applications maintain the olfactory stimulus and ensure that topical absorption continues.

Magnesium Lotion–Topical Nervous System Support

Magnesium chloride lotion or oil applied directly to the legs during a symptomatic episode provides both a potential direct magnesium delivery route and a mechanical calming effect through the act of firm self-massage. The evidence for transdermal magnesium absorption is less definitive than for oral magnesium, but the clinical experience among people with RLS who use it regularly is consistently positive—and the mechanism for local muscle relaxation through topical application of magnesium chloride to overactive tissue is physiologically plausible independent of systemic absorption questions.

Applied to both calves and shins with moderate pressure—firm enough to produce a slight warming sensation in the tissue—magnesium lotion provides a sensory input that partially competes with and interrupts the crawling or tingling sensation of RLS. This is not simply distraction; pressure and warmth activate mechanoreceptors in the skin and underlying tissue that send competing signals to the spinal cord and brainstem, partially gating the abnormal sensory signals that RLS generates.

Keep magnesium lotion on the bedside table alongside the essential oil roller. Apply it to both legs as a Tier 1 intervention, ideally in combination with breathwork and essential oils rather than as a sequential replacement for them. The combination of olfactory calming, topical essential oil absorption, and magnesium lotion mechanical stimulation creates a multi-channel sensory input that is more effective than any single approach alone.

Positional Changes and Pressure–Sensory Competition

Changing leg position in bed and applying deliberate pressure to the symptomatic areas exploits a neurological principle called sensory gating—the spinal cord's mechanism for prioritizing and filtering sensory signals. Intense, focused pressure in an area experiencing the crawling sensations of RLS temporarily saturates the sensory pathways with competing tactile information, reducing the brain's ability to process the RLS signal with the same intensity.

Practical techniques: pressing both hands firmly against the calves or shins for thirty to sixty seconds, using a firm pillow wedged tightly against the legs, lying on the side with the legs pressed together so one applies pressure to the other, or crossing the ankles and squeezing. Some people find that pulling the toes back firmly toward the shin (dorsiflexion) while pressing the heel into the mattress provides a few seconds of symptom interruption that creates enough of a window for breathwork to take hold.

These techniques do not address the underlying neurochemical cause, and their relief is brief—typically thirty seconds to a few minutes. Their value is as symptom interrupters that create a neurological window rather than as standalone solutions. Used in combination with breathwork and topical applications, they form part of a layered in-bed response that is often sufficient to allow symptoms to settle without requiring full movement.

Tier 2—Targeted Stretching and Self-Massage

If Tier 1 interventions have been attempted for five to ten minutes without adequate relief, moving to Tier 2 is the appropriate response.

These techniques involve sitting up in bed or standing at the bedside, but do not require leaving the sleep environment or turning on stimulating lights.

Targeted Stretching–Calf, Hamstring, and Hip Flexor Release

Stretching provides temporary but reliable relief from RLS symptoms through two mechanisms: It activates Golgi tendon organs—sensory receptors in the muscle-tendon junction that respond to stretch by triggering a reflexive inhibitory signal to the stretched muscle—and it temporarily increases local circulation to the legs, which may partially address the vascular component of the crawling sensation. Stretching does not resolve the underlying neurochemical cause, but it reliably interrupts the active symptom cycle for several minutes, which is often long enough for the Tier 1 interventions to consolidate their effect.

The most effective stretches for acute RLS relief, each held for 30 to 60 seconds per side:

- **Standing calf stretch:** Facing a wall, place both hands flat against it at shoulder height. Step one foot back approximately two feet, keeping the back heel flat on the floor and the knee straight. Lean the body forward gently until a firm stretch is felt in the back calf. Hold, breathe slowly, then switch sides. This directly addresses the calf—the most common site of RLS discomfort—and is one of the fastest-acting stretches for symptom interruption.
- **Seated hamstring stretch:** Sitting on the edge of the bed, extend one leg straight with the heel resting on the floor. Keeping the back straight, lean forward gently from the hips until a stretch is felt along the back of the thigh. Hold,

breathe, switch sides. Particularly useful when RLS sensations extend into the back of the thighs or when the calf stretch alone has not produced adequate relief.

- **Hip flexor lunge stretch:** Kneeling on one knee at the bedside with the other foot forward, gently press the hips forward until a stretch is felt at the front of the hip and upper thigh of the kneeling leg. The hip flexors connect to the lower back and pelvis in ways that can contribute to the referred restlessness sensations some people experience in the thighs and lower back alongside their RLS. This stretch is particularly relevant when discomfort extends above the knee.
- **Ankle rotations and dorsiflexion:** seated on the edge of the bed, rotate each ankle ten times in each direction, then flex and extend each foot ten times. Simple but underestimated—ankle mobility work activates the proprioceptive system in the lower legs and increases local circulation without requiring significant effort or full standing.

Self-Massage–Firm and Deliberate

Firm self-massage of the calves, shins, and feet performed in conjunction with or immediately following stretching extends the sensory competition effect and adds mechanical circulatory stimulation. Use both hands with moderate-to-firm pressure, working in long upward strokes from the ankle toward the knee on the calves, and using thumbs to apply targeted pressure to the arch and heel of each foot.

Applying the acute-relief essential oil blend during this massage delivers topical lavender and marjoram compounds while the mechanical stimulation of massage enhances skin absorption through increased local circulation. Two to three minutes of deliberate self-massage per leg—reapplying oil if needed—provides enough combined sensory, circulatory, and pharmacological input to interrupt most moderate-severity symptom episodes.

Tier 3–Active Relief When Symptoms Demand It

Some nights, particularly in the early weeks of the strategy before iron levels have improved, Tier 1 and 2 interventions are not enough. The symptoms are too severe or too persistent. When that is the case, getting up and moving is the right response—not a failure of the protocol, but an appropriate deployment of the most powerful short-term RLS interrupter available: movement.

The reason movement provides such reliable relief is neurological: walking activates the spinal central pattern generators—neural circuits in the spinal cord that coordinate rhythmic movement—and simultaneously suppresses the overactivated sensory pathways that generate RLS symptoms. The relief is typically rapid and complete during movement, though symptoms tend to return when movement stops. The goal of Tier 3 interventions is not prolonged activity but a strategic reset—enough movement to interrupt the symptom cycle and allow the nervous system to settle to a lower baseline before returning to bed.

Walking–Brief, Deliberate, and With Intention

Walking for relief from acute RLS does not need to be prolonged. Five to ten minutes of deliberate walking at a moderate pace—enough to feel the rhythmic activation of the leg muscles through their full range of motion—is usually sufficient to interrupt the episode and reset the nervous system's sensory baseline. Walking up and down a hallway, pacing slowly around a room, or walking up and down a flight of stairs all achieve the same effect.

The critical technique for sleep reinstatement after a walking bout is the management of the return to bed. After walking, avoid stimulating activities—do not check your phone, scroll social media, or turn on a television. Sit or lie in a dimly lit space, resume slow breathing, and allow a gradual return of drowsiness before lying down again. Returning to bed immediately while still alert from movement often leads to a repeat episode within minutes because the nervous system has not had time to settle. A five-minute transition of slow breathing in dim light after walking provides a more effective bridge back to sleep onset.

Temperature Therapy—Hot, Cold, and Contrast

Temperature application to the legs is one of the most effective and underused quick-relief strategies in the RLS toolkit. Both heat and cold provide meaningful symptom relief, and some people find that alternating between them—contrast therapy—is more effective than either alone. The mechanism differs for each:

- **Heat**—applied as a warm compress, heated pad, or warm bath or shower, increases local circulation and promotes muscle relaxation through thermal effects on muscle spindles. Many people with RLS find that warm water on the legs during a shower provides immediate, substantial relief—the warmth combined with the water pressure creates a strong sensory input that effectively overrides the RLS signal while the treatment is applied. The limitation of heat is that it tends to provide relief during and immediately after application, with symptoms sometimes returning within 20 to 30 minutes.

- **Cold**—applied as a cold pack, ice pack wrapped in a cloth, or cool water, activates cold thermoreceptors and A-delta nerve fibers in a way that strongly competes with the C-fiber sensory signals generating the RLS crawling sensation. Cold application is often faster-acting than heat for acute symptom interruption and can be maintained for longer periods. Applied to the calves and thighs for five to ten minutes, cold therapy can produce meaningful symptom relief that outlasts the application itself by 15 to 30 minutes in many people.
- **Contrast therapy**—alternating between warm and cool water during a shower, or between a warm compress and a cold pack, creates a pumping effect in peripheral circulation and activates multiple thermoreceptor populations simultaneously. Thirty seconds of warm followed by thirty seconds of cool, repeated four to five times per leg, is a practical protocol that many people find more effective than sustained application of either temperature alone. End on cool rather than warm for better sensory saturation and longer-lasting relief.

A practical nighttime implementation of temperature therapy that does not require a full shower: Keep a cold pack or a small container of ice in the freezer and a lightweight heating pad by the bed. This makes temperature therapy available without the alerting effect of a full bathroom trip and shower—particularly useful between Tier 2 and Tier 3 when symptoms need more than stretching but a full walk and shower feel excessive.

The Warm Bath or Shower–Full Symptom Reset

For severe episodes that have not responded to earlier interventions, a warm bath or shower—combined with essential oil application afterward—represents the most reliable full-reset available. Warm water on the legs and lower body activates mechanoreceptors and thermoreceptors across a wide surface area simultaneously, strongly suppressing the RLS sensory signal during the application. The core body temperature rise from a warm bath also triggers the rapid temperature drop that follows—the same drop that naturally facilitates sleep onset—making a warm bath 60 to 90 minutes before bed an effective sleep preparation strategy.

After a warm shower or bath, immediately apply the acute-relief essential oil blend to the legs while the skin is still warm and circulation is elevated—absorption is enhanced and the calming effect of the lavender-marjoram combination is amplified by the physiological state the warm water has created. Return to the sleep environment, resume breathwork, and allow the post-bath temperature drop to support sleep reinstatement.

What to Do When Symptoms Persist—Managing Difficult Nights

Some nights, particularly in the early weeks or during periods of high stress, illness, or significant iron depletion, symptoms persist despite working through the full toolkit. This is a real and valid experience that deserves an honest response rather than a reassuring platitude.

When a night goes badly despite a full toolkit response, the most important things to protect are the following morning's routines and the following night's protocol. Sleep deprivation from one bad night worsens the inflammatory environment, depletes magnesium through cortisol elevation, and impairs the adenosinergic wind-down the following evening—each of which can create a two-night cascade from a single difficult episode. Actively protecting the next day's practices—morning light, iron supplement if due, a nutrient-dense breakfast, an early caffeine cutoff, and especially the full evening protocol—breaks that cascade.

If a difficult night happens, resist the impulse to sleep late the following morning to compensate. While it feels restorative, sleeping significantly past the normal wake time disrupts the circadian anchor that the morning light protocol is building, making the following night's sleep and symptom picture worse rather than better. Getting up within 30 to 60 minutes of the normal wake time—even after a poor night—and getting immediate bright light exposure is the fastest way to stabilize the circadian clock and minimize the cascading effects of a bad night.

On nights when symptoms are already well-managed—which will increase in frequency as the protocol takes hold—the toolkit functions as a maintenance layer rather than a crisis response. A brief application of oil, a minute of slow breathing, and a couple of calf stretches before lying down each night keeps the system primed and the sensory environment well-managed even when the underlying biology is in good order.

> *The toolkit does not fail on a bad night—bad nights are data. They show which conditions worsen symptoms, which tools work best for your specific presentation, and how quickly the system recovers when the full protocol is reinstated the following day. Every difficult night is information you are gathering toward a better strategy.*

Quick Reference—The Tiered Response at a Glance

The following is a condensed reference for use in the moment, when consulting a full chapter is not practical. Post it on the bedside table or in a notes app on your phone until the sequence becomes automatic.

Tier 1—Try These First, Without Getting Up

- **Slow breathing:** 4 count inhale, 6 to 8 count exhale. Six to eight cycles.
- **Essential oil roller:** apply acute-relief blend to both calves and shins. Repeat in 5 to 10 minutes if needed.
- **Magnesium lotion:** apply with firm pressure to both legs.
- **Pressure and position change:** firm hand pressure on calves 30 to 60 seconds, change leg position, press legs together.

Tier 2—If Tier 1 Has Not Worked After 5 to 10 Minutes

- **Calf stretch:** 30 to 60 seconds per side at the bedside, with slow breathing throughout.
- **Hamstring stretch:** seated at the edge of the bed, one leg extended, 30 to 60 seconds per side.
- **Self-massage with oil:** firm upward strokes from ankle to knee, 2 to 3 minutes per leg, with oil reapplied.
- **Ankle rotations and dorsiflexion:** 10 circles each direction per ankle, 10 flex-extends per foot.

Tier 3—When Tier 2 Is Not Enough

- **Walk:** 5 to 10 minutes at a moderate pace. Follow with 5 minutes of slow breathing in dim light before returning to bed.
- **Cold pack to calves:** 5 to 10 minutes. Apply oil blend immediately after removal.

- **Contrast therapy:** alternating warm and cool on the legs, 30 seconds each, 4 to 5 cycles. End on cool.
- **Warm shower:** full reset. Apply essential oil blend immediately after. Resume breathwork. Allow 5 to 10 minutes before returning to bed.

What You Need to Take Away From This Chapter

- **The quick-relief toolkit is a layered system**, not a list of equivalent options. Start with the least disruptive interventions and escalate only when genuinely needed.
- **Breathwork is always the first response**—it is immediately available, costs nothing, and directly reduces the sympathetic overactivation that amplifies symptoms.
- **Bedside readiness matters**—having the acute-relief roller blend and magnesium lotion on the bedside table means Tier 1 tools are available without needing to get up, turn on lights, or prepare anything.
- **Temperature therapy is one of the most effective and underused tools**—cold application for fast-acting sensory competition, warm water for full-reset situations, and contrast therapy for extended relief.
- **After any Tier 3 intervention, manage the return to sleep deliberately**—five minutes of slow breathing in dim light before lying back down dramatically improves sleep reinstatement compared to going straight from walking or showering back to bed.
- **Bad nights are information**, not failures. Protect the next morning's routines to prevent the cascade effect, and use the data from difficult nights to refine the prevention strategy.

• • •

In Chapter 12, we address when the strategy calls for going deeper—the signs that advanced testing, specific investigation, or practitioner support is warranted, and how to approach those conversations with clarity.

CHAPTER TWELVE

WHEN TO DIG DEEPER

For many people, the strategy laid out in the preceding chapters—Restore, Deliver, Calm—will produce meaningful and durable improvement. Ferritin climbs, inflammation decreases, the nervous system begins to regulate more reliably, and nights become progressively more manageable. The framework, implemented consistently, is sufficient for the majority of people with RLS.

But not for everyone. Some people implement everything correctly, with genuine commitment and appropriate patience, and still find that progress stalls—ferritin refuses to move, symptoms remain severe despite months of careful effort, or a persistent pattern of improvement followed by regression suggests something is still unresolved beneath the surface. Others find that their symptoms do not fit the typical RLS picture cleanly, or that the co-occurring health issues in their picture are complex enough that self-directed management is insufficient.

This chapter is for those situations. It covers the signs that a deeper investigation is warranted, the specific tests and targets that provide the most useful clinical picture for RLS, and how to approach a conversation with a practitioner in a way that makes the most of that engagement. Knowing when to ask for more help—and what specifically to ask for—is not a concession that the natural approach has failed. It is the intelligent application of the same root-cause thinking that has guided this entire guide.

Signs That Deeper Investigation Is Warranted

The following situations represent genuine signals that something beyond the standard framework requires attention. They are not reasons for panic, but they are reasons to move from self-directed management to a more thorough clinical evaluation.

Ferritin Not Moving Despite Three to Four Months of Consistent Effort

Ferritin that remains stuck below 50 nanograms per milliliter after three to four months of well-implemented dietary optimization and supplementation—correct form, alternate-day dosing, proper timing, vitamin C pairing, and no obvious absorption blockers—is a signal that something specific is impairing absorption or creating an ongoing iron loss that supplementation alone cannot overcome.

The most common explanations include undiagnosed gut conditions such as celiac disease or *H. pylori* infection, an ongoing source of blood loss that has not been identified, a chronic inflammatory state maintaining hepcidin elevation despite dietary intervention, or a genetic variant affecting iron absorption. None of these is detectable without investigation. If ferritin is simply not moving, the appropriate response is not to try harder with the same approach—it is to find out why.

Symptoms That Are Severe, Daily, and Significantly Disabling

Severe RLS that affects every night, involves hours of disrupted sleep, and significantly impairs daytime functioning—cognitive performance, mood, occupational capacity, relationships—represents a quality-of-life impact that warrants clinical partnership rather than exclusively self-directed management. While the natural strategy in this guide can and does produce meaningful improvement even in severe cases, the timeline for iron restoration means the early months require adequate support.

For severe presentations, the natural strategy and clinical support are not mutually exclusive. A practitioner can provide intravenous iron to accelerate the restoration that oral supplementation would accomplish more slowly, evaluate for co-occurring conditions that require their own treatment, and—where medication is genuinely indicated as a bridge during acute severity—do so with a more informed picture of the full biological context than the standard prescribing model usually provides.

Symptoms That Do Not Follow the Classic RLS Pattern

The classic RLS pattern—worse at rest, partially relieved by movement, worse in the evening—is distinct enough that when symptoms deviate significantly from it, alternative diagnoses deserve consideration. Symptoms that are primarily present during exercise rather than rest, that are not relieved by movement, that involve significant pain rather than the crawling or tingling character of RLS, or that are associated with significant weakness or numbness may represent peripheral neuropathy, vascular insufficiency, or other neurological conditions that require their own diagnostic evaluation.

Getting a diagnosis confirmed—rather than assumed—also matters for treatment. The interventions in this guide are targeted at RLS specifically. If a significant proportion of the symptoms have a different etiology (the fundamental cause or origin of a condition or disease), those symptoms may not respond to the RLS framework regardless of how carefully it is implemented. A thorough clinical evaluation rules out other causes and focuses the strategy appropriately.

A Sudden Dramatic Worsening After a Period of Stability

Intermittent RLS that periodically worsens is expected and within the normal range of the condition. But a sudden, dramatic, unexplained worsening of symptoms—particularly in someone who has had stable or well-managed RLS—often signals that something specific has changed: A new medication has been introduced, an underlying health condition has developed or progressed, a significant nutritional depletion has occurred, or a new inflammatory trigger has emerged.

This pattern is worth investigating specifically rather than simply intensifying the general protocol. The most productive first step is a medication review—checking whether anything new has been added in the weeks prior to the worsening. SSRIs, antihistamines, antipsychotics, and proton pump inhibitors are all common culprits. If no medication change explains it, a comprehensive lab panel including iron markers, inflammatory markers, B12, folate, and thyroid function (TSH, free T4 and T3, TPOAb, TgAb, rT3, total T3, and FTI, with testing occurring in the early morning) provides the most useful diagnostic starting point.

RLS in Pregnancy

Pregnancy-related RLS deserves specific clinical attention for several reasons. The iron and folate demands of the developing baby create a rapidly changing nutritional picture that requires monitoring beyond what self-directed supplementation can reliably address. Some of the interventions in this guide—including certain essential oils and herbal compounds—carry pregnancy-specific cautions that make practitioner guidance more important, not less. And the severity of RLS in some pregnancies, combined with the sleep deprivation of the third trimester, creates a situation where the quality-of-life impact alone justifies professional support.

An obstetrician or midwife familiar with the iron-RLS connection can monitor ferritin and folate throughout the pregnancy and adjust supplementation based on changing needs—a level of responsive monitoring that self-directed management cannot replicate. Pregnancy-related RLS often resolves postpartum, but women who remain iron-depleted after delivery are at elevated risk for persistent symptoms and benefit from continued monitoring in the months following delivery.

Co-Occurring Conditions That Complicate the Picture

Certain co-occurring health conditions substantially complicate self-directed RLS management and benefit from integrated clinical support. These include chronic kidney disease (where iron metabolism is profoundly disrupted and standard oral supplementation is often ineffective); inflammatory bowel disease (where iron absorption is impaired and iron supplementation requires specific clinical management); active autoimmune conditions (where the inflammatory picture driving hepcidin elevation requires its own treatment); and significant mental health conditions (where the interaction between RLS, sleep, medications, and psychological wellbeing creates a complexity that benefits from clinical coordination).

In each of these situations, the natural strategy in this guide remains relevant and largely applicable, but the additional clinical layer is not optional. It is the responsible approach.

Advanced Testing—Going Beyond the Basic Iron Panel

The standard iron panel—serum iron, ferritin, and occasionally transferrin saturation—provides useful information but leaves significant gaps in the clinical picture for a challenging RLS case. The following tests represent the most informative additions to that baseline for someone whose situation warrants deeper investigation.

The Complete Iron Picture—Targets and Context

For RLS, the relevant iron markers and their meaningful targets are as follows:

- **Ferritin:** the target for RLS symptom improvement is 100 nanograms per milliliter or above. The range of 100 to 150 is where most people with RLS begin to experience meaningful, durable benefit. Levels of 75 to 100 represent a functional deficit by RLS standards even if the laboratory flags them as normal. Levels below 50 represent significant insufficiency requiring active correction. Levels above 200 warrant discussion with a clinician to rule out an inflammatory cause of ferritin elevation rather than genuine iron excess.
- **Transferrin saturation:** ideally between 25 and 35 percent. Below 20 percent alongside any ferritin level suggests impaired iron transport—hepcidin-mediated or

otherwise. Above 45 percent, particularly with elevated ferritin, may warrant further evaluation for hemochromatosis—a genetic iron overload condition.

- **Total iron-binding capacity (TIBC):** typically reported alongside transferrin saturation on standard iron panels, since transferrin saturation is calculated directly from serum iron divided by TIBC. TIBC reflects how much unoccupied iron-binding capacity exists in circulation—a high TIBC indicates the body is producing extra transferrin to capture more iron, which is a consistent signal of iron deficiency. A low TIBC alongside elevated ferritin and high transferrin saturation may suggest iron overload or inflammation suppressing transferrin production and warrants clinical discussion. For most people reviewing their results, TIBC is most useful as context for interpreting transferrin saturation rather than as an independently actionable number.
- **Serum iron:** useful in context but not reliably diagnostic alone. Serum iron fluctuates significantly throughout the day and between days, and should be interpreted alongside ferritin and transferrin saturation rather than in isolation.
- **C-reactive protein (CRP):** a low CRP—ideally below 1 milligram per liter—confirms that ferritin is reflecting genuine iron stores rather than inflammatory elevation. An elevated CRP alongside borderline ferritin is a signal that ferritin is being falsely elevated by inflammation and the true iron store picture may be worse than the ferritin number suggests.
- **Soluble transferrin receptor (sTfR):** a more specialized marker that reflects cellular iron demand at the tissue level. When cells are starved of iron, they upregulate transferrin receptors to capture more of what is circulating—sTfR rises as a measurable signal of that demand. Unlike ferritin, it is not elevated by inflammation, which makes it the most reliable marker for confirming functional iron deficiency when CRP is elevated and ferritin may be inflated by

inflammatory activity rather than genuine iron adequacy. One practical caution before interpreting a sTfR result: Reference ranges vary substantially between laboratories depending on which assay they use. Different commercial assays use different calibrators and antibodies, so results (and reference intervals) are not interchangeable across labs. Mayo Clinic Laboratories reports a reference range of 0.63–2.64 mg/L; other laboratories use ranges such as 0.76–1.76 mg/L or 0.8–1.7 mg/L; and some labs (like LabCorp) report in different units entirely (nmol/L rather than mg/L), making direct comparison impossible without knowing the specific assay. Always interpret sTfR against the reference range printed on your own laboratory's report rather than values found in other sources—the number means nothing without that context. Within your lab's reference range, the general interpretive framework is as follows. A result within the normal range suggests iron-deficient erythropoiesis (the biological process of producing new red blood cells in the bone marrow) is unlikely and tissue iron stores are adequate. A borderline elevated result—in the upper portion of or just above the reference range—suggests mild functional iron deficiency at the cellular level and warrants interpretation alongside ferritin and transferrin saturation together. A clearly elevated result indicates significant iron-deficient erythropoiesis and supports investigation for absolute or functional iron deficiency. The most clinically useful derived value is the sTfR/log ferritin ratio. A ratio above 2.0 confirms iron-deficient erythropoiesis regardless of what individual markers show in isolation. A ratio below 1.0 alongside elevated sTfR points instead toward anemia or chronic disease—a pattern in which iron stores are actually adequate but inflammation is preventing iron from being mobilized and used. This distinction matters directly for the RLS recovery strategy: The former calls for more aggressive iron restoration; the latter calls for prioritizing the Deliver phase inflammation reduction, since the iron is present but blocked, rather than absent. No RLS-specific sTfR thresholds have been established in the clinical literature. The interpretive values above are drawn from general iron metabolism frameworks. Their relevance to RLS lies in identifying which category of iron problem is present—absolute deficiency, functional restriction from inflammation, or adequacy—rather than in predicting symptom severity at a specific number.

> *When requesting a lab panel, ask for ferritin, transferrin saturation, serum iron, and CRP as a minimum. If inflammation is present or ferritin seems inconsistent with clinical symptoms, adding soluble transferrin receptor provides the most complete picture of actual iron availability at the cellular level.*

Gut-Related Testing—When Iron Refuses to Move

When ferritin fails to respond adequately to optimized oral supplementation, gut-related testing is the most productive next investigative step. The following represent the most useful options depending on clinical context:

- **Celiac antibody panel (tTG-IgA and total IgA):** Celiac disease is significantly underdiagnosed and is one of the most common causes of iron deficiency that does not respond to oral supplementation. It is a straightforward blood test that should be among the first investigations when iron status fails to improve. Note that the test requires ongoing gluten consumption to be accurate—a gluten-free diet implemented before testing will produce a false negative.

- ***H. pylori* testing:** available as a breath test, stool antigen test, or blood antibody test. *H. pylori* infection impairs iron absorption through multiple mechanisms and is extraordinarily common—estimated to be present in nearly half of the global population.[135,136] Breath or stool antigen testing is more reliable than blood antibody testing for confirming active infection. If this is a concern, see my blog *Eradicating H. pylori Naturally* at: https://authorscott.com/eradicating-h-pylori-naturally/.
- **Fecal occult blood test:** screens for blood loss in the gastrointestinal tract that is not visible. A positive result warrants further gastroenterological evaluation to identify the source. Chronic gastrointestinal micro-bleeding—from ulcers, polyps, hemorrhoids, or inflammatory bowel disease—can create a persistent iron drain that supplementation cannot keep pace with.
- **Comprehensive stool testing:** Advanced stool panels from specialist laboratories can assess microbiome composition, intestinal permeability markers, inflammatory markers specific to the gut, and digestive enzyme function. These are more expensive and more specialized than standard clinical tests, but for people with significant gut symptoms alongside their RLS, they provide a level of detail that standard clinical testing does not.

Nutrient and Metabolic Testing—Filling the Cofactor Picture

Beyond iron, the following nutrient tests are most directly relevant to the RLS root cause picture and most commonly overlooked in standard clinical workups:

- **25-hydroxyvitamin D:** the most accurate measure of vitamin D status. Target 50 to 80 nanograms per milliliter for optimal neurological and immune function. Below 30 represents clear deficiency; below 20 is severe deficiency requiring aggressive correction.

- **B12 and folate:** both assessed together for their combined relevance to neurological function and RLS. Active B12 (holotranscobalamin) is a more sensitive marker of true B12 status than total serum B12, particularly in older adults where transport protein abnormalities can make total B12 misleadingly normal.
- **Homocysteine:** Elevated homocysteine is a sensitive downstream signal that the methylation cycle—which depends on adequate B12, folate, and B6—is not functioning optimally, even when individual B vitamin levels appear normal on standard testing. It adds interpretive value that individual vitamins alone can miss. One specific reason homocysteine can remain elevated despite apparently adequate B vitamin intake is an MTHFR gene variant. MTHFR encodes the enzyme that converts dietary and supplemental folate into its biologically active form, 5-methyltetrahydrofolate (5-MTHF). The C677T and A1298C variants—which are common, with the C677T homozygous form present in roughly 10 to 15 percent of many populations—reduce this conversion efficiency significantly.[137,138,139,140] A person with a significant MTHFR variant can have normal or high serum folate while having functionally insufficient active folate at the cellular level, producing elevated homocysteine as the downstream signal of that gap. Standard folic acid supplementation, which requires the same impaired enzyme to become usable, will likely provide little benefit in this situation. Indeed, it may actually make the problem worse because unmetabolized folic acid may block folate receptors in the brain and kidneys.[141] Pre-methylated folate—sold as 5-MTHF or methylfolate—bypasses the conversion step entirely and is the appropriate form for people with meaningful MTHFR variants. Folinic acid (usually listed as 'calcium folinate' or

'folinic acid, calcium salt' on supplement labels) is also suitable for individuals who don't tolerate methylfolate—it can cause anxiety and overstimulation in some people—or need folate for DNA synthesis and tissue repair support. It sems to reduce homocysteine as well as methylfolate and in certain genotypes (C677T heterozygous) may perform even better;[142] however, in those with severe MTHFR impairment (e.g., TT homozygous) or additional pathway issues (e.g., MTHFS variants) folinic acid can be less than ideal due to conversion bottlenecks and accumulation. Methylcobalamin or adenosylcobalamin are similarly preferred over cyanocobalamin as B12 forms in this context. The RLS relevance extends beyond B vitamin status alone: the methylation cycle is required for dopamine synthesis and metabolism, connecting MTHFR-related methylation impairment directly to the dopaminergic picture underlying RLS. For anyone with persistently elevated homocysteine despite dietary optimization and standard B vitamin supplementation, MTHFR testing—available through standard genetic panels and consumer testing services—is a worthwhile next step that may change both the supplement forms and the clinical approach.

- **Red blood cell magnesium:** a more accurate reflection of intracellular magnesium status than serum magnesium, which—as discussed in Chapter 8—can appear normal while tissue stores are significantly depleted. Not available at all laboratories but worth requesting specifically in a challenging case.
- **Serum copper and ceruloplasmin:** For people in whom iron restoration is proceeding normally but RLS improvement is lagging, checking copper and its transport protein ceruloplasmin can identify the iron mobilization bottleneck discussed in Chapter 4.
- **Thyroid function (TSH, free T3, free T4, rT3, antibodies, and FTI):** Hypothyroidism is associated with

RLS through multiple mechanisms including impaired iron metabolism, reduced dopaminergic function, and peripheral neuropathy that can produce RLS-like symptoms. A full thyroid panel rather than TSH alone provides a more complete picture, as normal TSH with low free T3 can still represent functionally inadequate thyroid status.

- **Fasting glucose and insulin:** Insulin resistance and metabolic syndrome are associated with chronic inflammation, elevated hepcidin, and impaired iron delivery. For people with excess body weight, sedentary lifestyles, or a diet high in refined carbohydrates, assessing metabolic health is a relevant component of the inflammatory picture.

Genetic Testing—When Hereditary Patterns Are Present

For people with a strong family history of RLS, early onset of symptoms, or iron status that suggests hemochromatosis or other iron metabolism disorders, genetic testing provides information that changes the management picture.

HFE gene testing identifies the most common genetic variant associated with hereditary hemochromatosis—a condition of iron overload that, paradoxically, can in early stages coexist with functional brain iron deficiency while total body iron is elevated. Knowing carrier status for HFE variants changes the supplementation approach significantly and makes clinical supervision of iron restoration particularly important.

For RLS specifically, several gene variants in the BTBD9, MEIS1, MAP2K5, and PTPRD loci are associated with elevated RLS risk through mechanisms related to iron metabolism and dopaminergic function.[143] Consumer genetic testing services make this information accessible, but interpreting it meaningfully in a clinical context benefits from discussion with a practitioner familiar with the genetics-RLS relationship.

Working With a Practitioner—Getting the Most From Clinical Support

The quality of clinical support available for RLS varies considerably. Some neurologists, sleep medicine specialists, and integrative medicine practitioners are deeply familiar with the current iron-centered understanding of RLS and approach management accordingly. Others—including many general practitioners—are working from an older framework that treats RLS primarily as a dopamine deficiency problem and defaults to medication without meaningful investigation of root causes.

Going into clinical appointments informed and prepared makes an enormous difference. The following guidance is designed to help you have more productive clinical conversations regardless of the practitioner's level of RLS-specific expertise.

Choosing the Right Type of Practitioner

For straightforward iron assessment and management, a well-informed primary care physician can provide the necessary testing and support, particularly if they are open to the ferritin target range discussion and understand the limitations of standard reference ranges for RLS.

For more complex situations—severe or treatment-resistant RLS, significant co-occurring conditions, or a case where investigation has not identified the driving factor—the following specialist types offer the most relevant expertise:

- **Sleep medicine specialists:** are typically the most familiar with current RLS management, including the iron-brain connection, augmentation from dopamine agonists, and intravenous iron as a treatment option. A sleep medicine evaluation also assesses for PLMD and other sleep disorders that may be compounding the RLS picture.
- **Neurologists with movement disorder expertise:** particularly those who treat Parkinson's disease, are often most current on the dopaminergic and iron-related aspects of RLS, since the conditions share overlapping biology and have driven much of the same research.
- **Integrative or functional medicine practitioners:** tend to bring the most comprehensive root-cause orientation to RLS, with greater willingness to evaluate nutrient cofactors, gut function, inflammatory markers, and lifestyle factors alongside the conventional iron picture. Quality varies significantly in this field—look for practitioners with specific training and a structured, evidence-based approach.
- **Gastroenterologists:** specifically relevant if gut dysfunction is suspected as a primary driver of iron absorption failure, or if celiac disease, inflammatory bowel disease, or *H. pylori* investigation is warranted.
- **Nephrologists:** For people with chronic kidney disease, nephrology offers the most informed approach to the combined iron metabolism, uremic, and inflammatory picture that makes kidney disease-related RLS so challenging to manage.

Preparing for the Appointment–What to Bring

Arriving at a clinical appointment prepared makes the difference between a ten-minute consultation that produces a prescription and a more substantive conversation that results in meaningful investigation. The following preparation pays dividends regardless of the practitioner type:

- **Bring your actual lab numbers:** not just the summary report saying "normal" or "within range"—the actual numerical values, particularly ferritin and transferrin saturation. Know your numbers before the appointment and be prepared to discuss them in the context of RLS-specific thresholds rather than population reference ranges.
- **Document symptom severity and pattern:** a brief written summary of how often symptoms occur, their typical severity on a zero to ten scale, the time of onset, how long episodes last, what helps, and what makes them worse. This structured description is more useful to a clinician than a verbal account and ensures that symptom severity is accurately represented rather than minimized in the moment.
- **List all current medications and supplements:** including over-the-counter products, herbal supplements, and any sleep aids. The medication-RLS interaction list from Chapter 4 is worth reviewing before the appointment to identify any potential contributors to discuss.
- **Describe what you have already tried:** including what form of iron supplementation, at what dose, for how long, and what effect it produced. This prevents starting from scratch and communicates the degree to which the standard first-line approach has already been addressed.
- **Know what you are asking for:** rather than arriving with a general sense that something needs to change, come with specific requests—the ferritin target range you are working toward, the additional markers you would like assessed, the gut investigation you believe is warranted, or the IV iron referral you would like to discuss. Specific requests are more likely to produce specific outcomes.

> *The most productive clinical conversations about RLS are ones where the person comes prepared with numbers, documented severity, and specific questions.*

> *A clinician who might reflexively offer a prescription becomes a more collaborative partner when the person across the desk clearly understands the condition and is asking informed questions about root causes.*

Having the Ferritin Target Conversation

The most common point of friction in clinical conversations about RLS and iron is the ferritin target. A practitioner trained on standard reference ranges may look at a ferritin of 45 and tell you it is normal. You now know that for RLS, 45 is associated with significant symptom burden and that the clinically meaningful target is 100 or above. Having this conversation productively requires framing, not confrontation.

A useful framing: "I understand my ferritin is within the standard reference range, and I am not questioning that. What I have read in the RLS-specific research is that the threshold below which brain iron appears to affect RLS symptoms is around 75 to 100 nanograms per milliliter—considerably higher than the anemia-prevention threshold. I would like to work toward that range and monitor whether my symptoms change as ferritin rises. Is that something we can approach together?"

This framing acknowledges the clinician's expertise, does not dismiss standard ranges, and invites collaboration rather than positioning the conversation as adversarial. Most clinicians, when presented with a person who is informed, reasonable, and asking for evidence-based support rather than demanding medication, respond constructively.

If a clinician is genuinely unfamiliar with the RLS-specific ferritin research, it is entirely appropriate to mention that the current guidelines from the International Restless Legs Syndrome Study Group address this distinction. This is not a confrontation—it is providing context that the clinician may not have had occasion to review recently. Most will appreciate the information.

When to Seek a Second Opinion

If a clinical appointment results in a medication prescription without any investigation of iron status, dismissal of iron as a relevant factor, refusal to order the tests that seem clinically warranted, or a response that does not engage meaningfully with the questions asked—a second opinion is not only reasonable but appropriate. Medical practice has significant variation, and RLS is an area where the gap between current evidence and standard practice remains wide in many clinical settings.

A second opinion is not an accusation that the first clinician was wrong—it is a recognition that complex conditions benefit from multiple informed perspectives, and that clinical expertise in RLS specifically is not uniformly distributed. Anyone with severe or treatment-resistant RLS deserves access to a clinician who is current on the science. If that requires seeking a specialist or a second appointment, that investment is worth making.

When Natural Approaches Need a Medical Partner

This guide has been clear throughout that the goal is root-cause resolution rather than symptom management, and that the natural strategy—when properly implemented—is sufficient for most people with RLS. But it would be intellectually dishonest to close the clinical chapter without acknowledging that there are situations in which the natural approach requires a medical partner to function optimally and situations in which medication plays a legitimate and carefully chosen role.

Intravenous iron is the clearest example. It is not a pharmaceutical treatment in the conventional sense—it is a targeted delivery method for the same intervention that lies at the heart of the natural strategy, bypassing the absorption limitations that can make oral restoration insufficient in severe cases. For the person with a ferritin of 18 and nightly symptoms that are clinically disabling, IV iron is not a concession to modern medicine—it is a faster and more direct path to the same destination.

Short-term pharmacological support—used as a bridge during the early months of iron restoration, with full awareness of its limitations and augmentation risks, in the smallest effective dose for the shortest effective period—can be a legitimate and rational choice for severe presentations where the quality-of-life impact of untreated RLS causes its own compounding harm. The person who cannot function, cannot maintain employment, or is developing serious secondary health consequences from months of severe sleep deprivation does not need to categorically refuse pharmaceutical support while waiting for ferritin to climb. They need a thoughtful, informed clinical partner who understands both the long-term strategy and the immediate situation.

The natural strategy and medical support are not opposing philosophies. They are tools in the same toolbox, applicable to different aspects of the same situation, used in the proportions that the individual case warrants.

What You Need to Take Away From This Chapter

- **Deeper investigation is warranted when ferritin is not responding, symptoms are severely disabling, the clinical pattern is atypical, or co-occurring conditions complicate the picture.** Recognizing these signals and acting on them is not giving up on the natural approach—it is applying the same root-cause logic with greater investigative depth.
- **The RLS-specific ferritin target is 100 nanograms per milliliter or above**—meaningfully higher than standard reference ranges. Knowing this number and advocating for it in clinical conversations is one of the most important pieces of information in this guide.
- **Advanced testing adds crucial layers beyond the basic iron panel**—soluble transferrin receptor, CRP, gut-related testing for celiac and *H. pylori*, nutrient cofactors, thyroid function, and metabolic markers provide the comprehensive picture that challenging cases require.
- **Prepared, specific, collaborative clinical conversations produce better outcomes** than vague complaints or passive receipt of a prescription. Arriving with numbers, documented severity, and specific requests changes the nature of the appointment.
- **Natural approaches and medical support are not mutually exclusive.** Intravenous iron, short-term pharmaceutical bridging when genuinely indicated, and specialist collaboration are all tools that serve the same goal: restoring the brain iron status and neurochemical balance that allows this condition to resolve.

• • •

In the Conclusion, we bring the full journey together—and remind you of what is now possible.

CHAPTER THIRTEEN

YOU ARE NOT STUCK WITH THIS

There is a particular kind of exhaustion that comes not just from lost sleep but from being dismissed. From having described something real and been told it was not that serious. From watching doctors reach for a prescription pad rather than ask what might actually be wrong. From lying awake night after night wondering whether this is simply how the rest of your life is going to feel.

If any of that resonates, then what you now hold is something more than a collection of interventions. It is a different story about what is happening in your body—one grounded in current science, respectful of your experience, and oriented toward resolution rather than indefinite management.

RLS is not random. It is not a character flaw or an exaggeration or an inevitable sentence. It is a biological signal—your nervous system communicating, loudly and persistently, that something specific is out of balance. The brain needs iron it is not receiving. The inflammatory environment is blocking delivery. The neurochemical systems that should quiet the evening are running short of what they need. These are not mysteries. They are identifiable, addressable, and in most cases correctable with the right approach applied with appropriate patience.

What Has Actually Changed

Before you encountered this material, RLS may have felt like something that happened to you—an unpredictable, uncontrollable nightly assault with no clear cause and no reliable solution. That is what the conventional experience of this condition often produces: a sense of helplessness that is itself a form of suffering layered on top of the physical symptoms.

Understanding the biology changes that experience in a fundamental way. When you know why your legs are restless—why the evening is worse, why movement helps, why certain medications create short-term relief and long-term problems—you are no longer a passive recipient of symptoms. You are someone who understands the mechanism and has specific, targeted tools for addressing it. That shift from helplessness to agency is not trivial. It is, for many people, one of the most meaningful things that comes from this kind of education.

You now know that brain iron deficiency is the root of the problem for most people—and that the ferritin number your doctor called normal may represent a genuine functional deficit by the standards of your brain's needs. You know that inflammation is not a vague background concern but a specific, measurable obstacle to iron delivery that can be reduced through concrete daily choices. You know that the nervous system overactivation driving your symptoms is not a permanent state but a correctable imbalance—one that responds to specific nutritional, lifestyle, and sensory inputs.

Most importantly, you know that the absence of a prescription is not the absence of a plan. There is a strategy here—coherent, sequenced, and grounded in the same science that should be informing clinical practice, whether or not it always does.

The Body's Remarkable Capacity to Recover

One of the most consistent observations among people who have implemented a genuine root-cause approach to RLS is the degree to which recovery seems to gather momentum over time. The first weeks are often the most difficult—the foundational work is underway but its effects are not yet visible, and the Calm phase tools are doing what they can against a nervous system that is still operating with a significant biological deficit.

Then something shifts. It is usually gradual rather than dramatic—a night here where symptoms arrives later than usual, a week where the toolkit is less frequently needed, a month where the pattern of dread around bedtime begins to ease. Ferritin numbers moving in the right direction. Sleep that, for the first time in years, is starting to feel like genuine rest rather than a nightly ordeal.

The nervous system is not fragile. Given the resources it has been depleted of and the space to recalibrate, it recovers. The brain's dopamine regulation systems, the GABA pathways, the adenosinergic wind-down mechanisms—these are not permanently damaged in the vast majority of people with RLS. They are undernourished and overloaded. Feed them what they need, reduce what is overloading them, and the system tends to right itself in ways that can feel almost surprising after years of it going in the wrong direction.

This is not a promise that every person will achieve complete resolution. Some presentations are more complex, some underlying conditions more persistent, some iron deficits deeper and harder to correct. But the direction of change—when the right inputs are applied consistently—is reliably toward improvement for the great majority of people who commit to this approach. The question is not usually whether it will work, but how carefully it is implemented and how long it will take.

> *Recovery from RLS is not a linear graph that moves only upward. It is a trend—an overall direction that, over months, bends toward better nights, more reliable sleep, and a life less organized around managing symptoms. The bad nights become less frequent. The good nights become the new normal.*

Beyond the Symptoms—What Recovery Actually Restores

RLS does not take only sleep. It takes the things that depend on sleep—the energy for the things that matter, the cognitive clarity to think, create, and engage, the emotional resilience to navigate a life fully rather than spending emotional reserves just getting through the night. It takes the freedom to travel, to sit through a dinner without fidgeting and apologizing, to be present in an evening with people you love without the private dread of what is coming when you lie down.

These are not small things. And they are exactly what becomes available again as this condition is brought under meaningful control.

There is also something worth naming about the broader changes that implementing this strategy tends to produce. The dietary patterns, the anti-inflammatory practices, the attention to gut health and nutrient sufficiency, the sleep optimization and stress management—none of these are isolated to RLS. They support the entire biological infrastructure of health. People who implement this approach for their legs often find, months in, that other things have quietly improved as well: energy levels, mood stability, digestive comfort, focus, resilience. The strategy that addresses RLS addresses far more than RLS.

A Final Word on Patience

The most difficult thing this guide asks of you is not the dietary changes or the supplement protocols or the evening routine. It is patience. It is the willingness to commit to a direction of change, the full benefit of which unfolds over months rather than days, and to hold that commitment through the nights when progress feels distant.

That patience is easier to sustain when it is grounded in understanding. When you know why ferritin takes months to rise, you can hold the strategy through a frustrating eighth week without concluding it is not working. When you understand why the nervous system does not recalibrate overnight, you can interpret a difficult night not as failure but as a data point in a longer arc that is moving in the right direction.

Understanding is not passive. It is, in the context of a condition that has been so persistently misunderstood and mismanaged, one of the most active and powerful things you can bring to your own recovery.

You came to this guide carrying something real—a condition that has disrupted your sleep, constrained your life, and too often been met with inadequate responses. You are leaving it with something real in return: a clear picture of what is actually happening, a coherent strategy for addressing it, and the knowledge that the experience of lying down without dread is not just a vague hope. For most people who do this work, it is what is waiting on the other side.

Your body is not broken. It is signaling. Now you know how to answer.

• • •

APPENDIX

THE 7-DAY RLS RESET PLAN

This appendix is a practical quick-start guide. It is not a replacement for the full strategy in the preceding chapters—the science, the sequencing, and the reasoning behind each intervention matter for long-term success. But this plan gives you a concrete place to begin: seven days of structured daily practice that introduce the most impactful elements of the Restore, Deliver, and Calm phases in a manageable, progressive sequence.

A few things to know before you start. First, this is a foundation week, not a transformation week. The goal is not to produce dramatic results in seven days—it is to establish the habits and routines that will produce meaningful results over the weeks and months that follow. Some people notice improvement in sleep quality and symptom severity within the first week, particularly from the Calm phase interventions. Others notice little change this early. Both are normal. Second, do not aim for perfection. Missing an item on a given day does not restart the clock. Progress is built through consistent direction over time, not flawless adherence to a checklist.

Read through the full seven-day plan before beginning so you can gather the supplies you need and have everything ready. The supply list at the end of this appendix covers everything required to implement the plan from day one.

What You Will Need Before You Begin

Supplements

- **Ferrous bisglycinate**—25 to 65 mg elemental iron per dose (confirm on label)
- **Vitamin C**—250 mg tablets or powder for pairing with iron
- **Magnesium glycinate**—200 to 400 mg elemental magnesium per dose
- **Glycine powder**—plain powder form; 3 to 5 g per serving
- **Taurine capsules or powder**—500 mg to 2 g per dose
- **Omega-3 fish oil or algae oil**—providing 1,000 to 2,000 mg combined EPA + DHA per dose
- **Vitamin D3 with K2**—2,000 to 4,000 IU D3 per dose

Essential Oils and Topicals

- **Lavender essential oil**—*Lavandula angustifolia*, quality tested (see Chapter 9 for sourcing guidance)
- **Carrier oil**—fractionated coconut oil, sweet almond oil, or jojoba
- **A 10-milliliter roller bottle**—available at health stores or online
- **Magnesium chloride lotion or oil**—for topical leg application
- **Optional diffuser**—ultrasonic, 100 milliliter capacity or larger

Practical Items

- **A light therapy lamp**—10,000 lux, if natural morning light is limited
- **Blue-light-blocking glasses**—amber-tinted lenses for evening screen use (Gunnar is a reputable brand)
- **A small notebook or phone notes app**—for the nightly tracking log

Before day one, prepare your roller blend: Add 10 drops of lavender essential oil to your 10-milliliter roller bottle and fill with carrier oil. Cap and roll between your palms to combine. Label it and place it on your bedside table.

The Daily Plans

Each day is organized into morning, midday, evening, and bedtime windows. New practices are introduced gradually across the week—items marked as NEW on each day are being added for the first time. Items from previous days carry forward automatically.

Day 1 Laying the Foundation

Day 1 focuses on the two practices with the largest immediate impact: morning light and the evening calming protocol. Keep everything else simple.

Morning

- ☐ Get outside or sit by a bright window within 60 minutes of waking—10 to 20 minutes (NEW)
- ☐ Take omega-3 with breakfast (NEW)
- ☐ Take vitamin D3 + K2 with breakfast (NEW)

Midday

- ☐ Have your last coffee, tea, or caffeinated soda before noon (NEW)
- ☐ Include protein in lunch—any animal source (NEW)

Evening—90 Minutes Before Bed

- ☐ Take magnesium glycinate (NEW)
- ☐ Mix 3 to 5 g glycine powder in water and drink (NEW)

- □ Shift to warm, dimmed lighting throughout the home (NEW)

Evening—60 Minutes Before Bed

- □ Apply lavender roller blend to both calves and shins—2 to 3 minutes per leg (NEW)
- □ Practice 4-7-8 or box breathing for 3 minutes (NEW)

Bedtime

- □ Cool the bedroom to 65 to 68°F (18 to 20°C) if possible
- □ Eliminate light sources in the sleeping environment
- □ Nightly log: note symptom severity (0 to 10) and sleep quality (0 to 10) (NEW)

Day 2 Adding Iron and Taurine

Day 2 introduces iron supplementation and taurine. Keep everything from Day 1 in place.

Morning—Before Breakfast

- □ Take ferrous bisglycinate with 250 mg vitamin C on an empty stomach (NEW)
- □ Wait at least 60 minutes before coffee
- □ Get morning light—10 to 20 minutes

Morning—With Breakfast

- □ Take omega-3
- □ Take vitamin D3 + K2

Midday

- □ Caffeine cutoff at noon
- □ Nutrient-dense lunch—protein, colorful vegetables, quality fat

Evening—90 Minutes Before Bed

- ☐ Take magnesium glycinate
- ☐ Take taurine—500 mg to 2 g (NEW)
- ☐ Mix glycine in water and drink
- ☐ Shift to dimmed, warm lighting
- ☐ Enable night mode on all screens

Evening—60 Minutes Before Bed

- ☐ Apply lavender roller blend to both legs
- ☐ Low-arousal activity—reading, calm music, light conversation (NEW)
- ☐ Breathwork—3 to 5 minutes

Bedtime

- ☐ Cool, dark sleeping environment
- ☐ Nightly log

Day 3 Rest Day for Iron—Gut and Inflammation Focus

Iron supplementation is taken on alternate days. Today the focus shifts to Deliver phase practices—anti-inflammatory food and gut support.

Morning

- ☐ Morning light—10 to 20 minutes
- ☐ Protein-rich breakfast—include a fermented food if available (yogurt, kefir, sauerkraut) (NEW)
- ☐ Omega-3 with breakfast
- ☐ Vitamin D3 + K2 with breakfast
- ☐ No iron supplement today (alternate-day rest)

Midday

- ☐ Caffeine cutoff at noon
- ☐ Include fatty fish at lunch or dinner today if possible (NEW)

- □ 20 to 30 minutes of moderate movement—walking, cycling, or similar (NEW)
- □ Include a variety of colorful vegetables at lunch

Evening—90 Minutes Before Bed

- □ Magnesium glycinate
- □ Taurine
- □ Glycine in water
- □ Dimmed, warm lighting

Evening—60 Minutes Before Bed

- □ Apply lavender roller blend to both legs
- □ Low-arousal activity
- □ Breathwork—3 to 5 minutes

Bedtime

- □ Cool, dark sleeping environment
- □ Nightly log—note any difference in symptoms compared to previous nights

Day 4 Iron Day—Adding Magnesium Lotion

Iron supplementation resumes today. A topical magnesium layer is added to the evening routine.

Morning—Before Breakfast

- □ Ferrous bisglycinate + 250 mg vitamin C on an empty stomach
- □ Wait 60 minutes before coffee
- □ Morning light

Morning—With Breakfast

- □ Omega-3
- □ Vitamin D3 + K2
- □ Include a fermented food at breakfast or lunch

Midday

- □ Caffeine cutoff at noon
- □ Nutrient-dense lunch with protein and colorful vegetables
- □ 20 to 30 minutes of moderate movement

Evening–90 Minutes Before Bed

- □ Magnesium glycinate
- □ Taurine
- □ Glycine in water
- □ Dimmed, warm lighting and screen night mode

Evening–60 Minutes Before Bed

- □ Apply lavender roller blend to both legs (now routine)
- □ Apply magnesium lotion to both calves with firm pressure (NEW)
- □ Low-arousal activity
- □ Breathwork—3 to 5 minutes

Bedtime

- □ Cool, dark sleeping environment
- □ Nightly log

Day 5 Rest Day for Iron—Deepening the Evening Routine

No iron supplement today. Focus on refining and deepening the evening protocol—adding the diffuser if available.

Morning

- □ Morning light
- □ Protein-rich breakfast with fermented food
- □ Omega-3 and vitamin D3 + K2 with breakfast
- □ No iron supplement today

Midday

- ☐ Caffeine cutoff at noon
- ☐ Include fatty fish at a meal today
- ☐ 20 to 30 minutes of moderate movement—complete by early afternoon if possible
- ☐ Brief stress reset: 5 minutes of slow breathing or a short outdoor walk at some point during the day (NEW)

Evening–90 Minutes Before Bed

- ☐ Magnesium glycinate
- ☐ Taurine
- ☐ Glycine in water
- ☐ Start bedroom diffuser with lavender blend—5 to 7 drops in 100 ml water (NEW if diffuser available)
- ☐ Dimmed, warm lighting throughout home
- ☐ Blue-light-blocking glasses on if using screens

Evening–60 Minutes Before Bed

- ☐ Apply lavender roller blend to both legs
- ☐ Apply magnesium lotion to calves
- ☐ Low-arousal activity—aim to avoid news and social media in this window
- ☐ Breathwork—3 to 5 minutes, before symptoms arrive

Bedtime

- ☐ Cool, dark sleeping environment
- ☐ If symptoms are present as you lie down—use Tier 1 tools before getting up
- ☐ Nightly log

Day 6 Iron Day—Full Protocol in Place

By Day 6, the core protocol is fully assembled. Today is about executing it with confidence and beginning to notice the direction of change.

Morning–Before Breakfast

- ☐ Ferrous bisglycinate + 250 mg vitamin C on an empty stomach
- ☐ Wait 60 minutes before coffee
- ☐ Morning light

Morning–With Breakfast

- ☐ Omega-3
- ☐ Vitamin D3 + K2
- ☐ Protein-anchored breakfast—include liver if this is one of your one to two times this week
- ☐ Fermented food at breakfast or lunch

Midday

- ☐ Caffeine cutoff at noon
- ☐ Varied, colorful lunch with protein and quality fat
- ☐ 20 to 30 minutes of moderate movement
- ☐ Brief midday decompression practice

Afternoon

- ☐ Dinner completed 2 to 3 hours before bed—protein-based with magnesium-rich vegetables
- ☐ Begin reducing cognitive and emotional stimulation 2 hours before the wind-down window

Evening–90 Minutes Before Bed

- ☐ Magnesium glycinate
- ☐ Taurine
- ☐ Glycine in water

- □ Bedroom diffuser started
- □ Dimmed lighting, blue-light-blocking glasses

Evening–60 Minutes Before Bed

- □ Lavender roller blend applied to both legs—3 to 5 minutes total
- □ Magnesium lotion applied with firm pressure
- □ Low-arousal activity only
- □ Breathwork—3 to 5 minutes

Bedtime

- □ Cool, dark sleeping environment
- □ Consistent bedtime—within 30 minutes of last night
- □ Nightly log

Day 7 Rest Day for Iron—Reflect and Plan Forward

The final day of the reset week. No iron supplement today. Take stock of how the week went and set intentions for the weeks ahead.

Morning

- □ Morning light
- □ Protein-rich breakfast with fermented food
- □ Omega-3 and vitamin D3 + K2
- □ No iron supplement today

Midday

- □ Caffeine cutoff at noon
- □ Movement—today's session can be slightly longer or more enjoyable if energy allows
- □ Take 10 minutes to review this week's nightly log—note any patterns, improvements, or items to refine

Afternoon

- ☐ Schedule your first ferritin blood test—8 weeks from now, to include ferritin, transferrin saturation, and CRP
- ☐ Prepare a fresh roller bottle blend if the current one is running low

Evening–90 Minutes Before Bed

- ☐ Magnesium glycinate
- ☐ Taurine
- ☐ Glycine in water
- ☐ Bedroom diffuser
- ☐ Dimmed lighting and blue-light-blocking glasses

Evening–60 Minutes Before Bed

- ☐ Lavender roller blend applied to both legs
- ☐ Magnesium lotion
- ☐ Low-arousal activity
- ☐ Breathwork—3 to 5 minutes

Bedtime

- ☐ Cool, dark sleeping environment
- ☐ Consistent bedtime
- ☐ Nightly log—Day 7 entry: Write one sentence about how this week compared to the week before

• • •

Weekly Habit Tracker

Use the table below to track completion of the core daily practices across the week. Check each box as each practice is completed. At the end of the week, any practice with five or more completed days represents a solid foundation. Items with fewer than four completed days are the priority focus for week two.

Practice	D1	D2	D3	D4	D5	D6	D7
Morning light (within 60 min of waking)	☐	☐	☐	☐	☐	☐	☐
Iron supplement (alternate days: 1, 3, 5, 7 = off)	☐	☐	☐	☐	☐	☐	☐
Omega-3 with breakfast	☐	☐	☐	☐	☐	☐	☐
Vitamin D3 + K2 with breakfast	☐	☐	☐	☐	☐	☐	☐
Caffeine cutoff at noon	☐	☐	☐	☐	☐	☐	☐
Protein-anchored lunch	☐	☐	☐	☐	☐	☐	☐
Fermented food at a meal	☐	☐	☐	☐	☐	☐	☐
20-40 min moderate movement	☐	☐	☐	☐	☐	☐	☐
Magnesium glycinate (90 min before bed)	☐	☐	☐	☐	☐	☐	☐
Glycine + taurine (evening)	☐	☐	☐	☐	☐	☐	☐
Dimmed lighting and screen management	☐	☐	☐	☐	☐	☐	☐
Lavender roller blend applied to legs	☐	☐	☐	☐	☐	☐	☐

Magnesium lotion applied to legs	☐	☐	☐	☐	☐	☐	☐
Breathwork—3 to 5 minutes	☐	☐	☐	☐	☐	☐	☐
Cool, dark sleeping environment	☐	☐	☐	☐	☐	☐	☐
Consistent bedtime	☐	☐	☐	☐	☐	☐	☐
Nightly log completed	☐	☐	☐	☐	☐	☐	☐

Daily Supplement and Oil Reference Card

Keep this reference in a visible location—on the bathroom mirror, the kitchen counter, or photographed on your phone—until the routine is automatic.

Morning–Before Breakfast (Alternate Days: Days 1, 3, 5, 7 Are Iron-Free)

- **Ferrous bisglycinate:** 25 to 65 mg elemental iron with 250 mg vitamin C. Wait 60 minutes before coffee.

Morning–With Breakfast (Daily)

- **Omega-3:** 1,000 to 2,000 mg EPA + DHA with a fat-containing meal
- **Vitamin D3 + K2:** 2,000 to 4,000 IU D3 with 100 mcg MK-7 K2, with a fat-containing meal

Evening–90 Minutes Before Bed (Daily)

- **Magnesium glycinate:** 200 to 400 mg elemental magnesium

- **Glycine:** 3 to 5 g dissolved in water
- **Taurine:** 500 mg to 2 g
- **Bedroom diffuser:** 5 to 7 drops lavender in 100 ml water—run 30 to 60 minutes

Evening–60 Minutes Before Bed (Daily)

- **Lavender roller blend:** applied to both calves, shins, and soles of feet—3 to 5 minutes total
- **Magnesium lotion:** applied with firm pressure to both calves

Acute Relief (As Needed)

- **Acute-relief roller:** lavender + marjoram + rosemary blend—apply to legs at first sign of symptoms
- **Breathwork:** 4 count inhale, 6 to 8 count exhale—6 to 8 cycles before escalating

• • •

Nightly Symptom and Sleep Log

Record entries each morning about the previous night. Two minutes is all it takes. The log will become a meaningful data record that shows progress over weeks and helps identify patterns.

Night	Symptom (0–10)	Sleep Quality (0–10)	Tool Used?	Notes (timing, deviations, observations)
Night 1				
Night 2				
Night 3				
Night 4				
Night 5				
Night 6				
Night 7				

After Day 7—What Comes Next

The 7-Day Reset establishes the core daily structure of the Restore, Deliver, and Calm phases. From Day 8 onward, the goal is to maintain and deepen what has been built—not to add more complexity, but to execute the existing protocol with increasing consistency and precision.

The practices most worth adding in weeks two and three, if not yet included, are a dedicated anti-inflammatory dietary shift (reducing ultra-processed foods and seed oils, increasing fatty fish and colorful vegetables), a probiotic or consistent fermented food daily, and curcumin if inflammatory markers are a concern. Chapter 7 covers each of these in detail.

Keep the nightly log going beyond Day 7. A running log over eight to twelve weeks—aligned with your first ferritin retest—provides the most informative picture of how the strategy is working and where to focus refinement. Improvement will not always be linear, but the trend over weeks will be visible in the numbers in a way that nightly impression alone often is not.

> *The 7-Day Reset is not the strategy—it is the first week of the strategy. What you have built in these seven days is a launchpad, not a destination. The improvement you are working toward unfolds over months, and the daily habits you have just established are what make those months productive.*

• • •

REFERENCES

[1] Song P, Wu J, Cao J, et al. The global and regional prevalence of restless legs syndrome among adults: A systematic review and modelling analysis. *J Glob Health*. 2024 Jun 7;14:04113.

[2] Abus S, Kapici Y, Ayhan S, et al. Elevated Cardiovascular Disease Risk in Patients with Restless Legs Syndrome. *Alpha Psychiatry*. 2023 May 1;24(3):95–99.

[3] Dunietz GL, Lisabeth LD, Shedden K, et al. Restless Legs Syndrome and Sleep-Wake Disturbances in Pregnancy. *J Clin Sleep Med*. 2017 Jul 15;13(7):863–870.

[4] Ghanei Gheshlagh R, Farajzadeh M, Zarei M, et al. The Prevalence of Restless Legs Syndrome in Patients Undergoing Hemodialysis: A Systematic Review and Meta-analysis Study. *Basic Clin Neurosci*. 2017 Mar-Apr;8(2):105–112.

[5] Allen RP, Picchietti DL, Garcia-Borreguero D, et al. Restless legs syndrome/Willis–Ekbom disease diagnostic criteria: updated International Restless Legs Syndrome Study Group (IRLSSG) consensus criteria—history, rationale, description, and significance. *Sleep Med*. 2014 Aug;15(8):860–873.

[6] Jimenez-Jimenez FJ, Alonso-Navarro H, Garcia-Martin E, et al. Association between restless legs syndrome and peripheral neuropathy: A systematic review and meta-analysis. *Eur J Neurol*. 2021 Jul;28(7):2423-42.

[7] An T, Sun H, Yuan L, Wu X, Lu B. Associations of anxiety and depression with restless legs syndrome: a systematic review and meta-analysis. *Front Neurol*. 2024 Mar 18;15:1366839.

[8] Marey H, Chai A, Bikow A. Periodic limb movements in sleep in patients using antidepressants. *Sleed Med Rev*. 2025 Feb;79:102011.

[9] Winkelman JW, Berkowski JA, DelRosso LM, et al. Treatment of restless legs syndrome and periodic limb movement disorder: an American Academy of Sleep Medicine clinical practice guideline. *J Clin Sleep Med*. 2025 Jan 1;21(1):137–152.

[10] Hornyak M, Feige B, Voderholzer U, Riemann D. Periodic leg movements in sleep and periodic limb movement disorder: prevalence, clinical significance and treatment. *Sleep Med Rev*. 2006 Oct;10(3):169–177.

[11] Montplaisir J, Boucher S, Poirier G, et al. Clinical, polysomnographic, and genetic characteristics of restless legs syndrome: a study of 133 patients diagnosed with new standard criteria. *Movement Disorders*. 1997 Jan;12(1):61–5.

[12] Garcia-Borreguero D, Silber MH, Winkelman JW, et al. Guidelines for the first-line treatment of restless legs syndrome/Willis–Ekbom disease: an IRLSSG task force report. *Sleep Med*. 2016 Jan;21:1–11.

[13] Beard JL, Connor JR. Iron status and neural functioning. *Annu Rev Nutr*. 2003;23:41–58.

[14] LeWitt PA. Levodopa therapy for Parkinson's disease: pharmacokinetics and pharmacodynamics. *Mov Disord*. 2015 Jan;30(1):64–72.

[15] Erikson KM, Jones BC, Beard JL. Iron deficiency alters dopamine transporter functioning in rat striatum. *J Nutr*. 2000 Nov;130(11):2831–2837.

[16] Earley CJ, Connor JR, Beard JL, et al. Abnormalities in CSF concentrations of ferritin and transferrin in restless legs syndrome. *Neurology*. 2000 May 23;54(10):1698–1700.

[17] Moos T, Morgan EH. The metabolism of neuronal iron and its pathogenic role in neurological disease: review. *Ann N Y Acad Sci.* 2004 Jun;1012:14–26.
[18] Schormair B, Kemlink D, Roeske D, et al. PTPRD (protein tyrosine phosphatase receptor type delta) is associated with restless legs syndrome. *Nat Genet.* 2008 Aug;40(8):946–948.
[19] Schormair B, Zhao C, Bell S, et al. Genome-wide meta-analyses of restless legs syndrome yield insights into genetic architecture, disease biology and risk prediction. *Nature Genetics.* 2024;56:1090-99.
[20] Allen RP, Barker PB, Wehrl F, Song HK, Earley CJ. MRI measurement of brain iron in patients with restless legs syndrome. *Neurology.* 2001 Aug 28;57(4):647–652.
[21] Anguizola D, Aragon AG, Moncada B, et al. Restless Legs Syndrome: Neurochemistry and Therapy. *Semin Neurol.* 2025 May;45(3):368-382.
[22] Ferré S, García-Borreguero D, Allen RP, Earley CJ. New insights into the neurobiology of restless legs syndrome. *Neuroscientist.* 2019 Feb;25(2):113–125.
[23] Anguizola D, Aragon AG, Moncada B, et al. Restless Legs Syndrome: Neurochemistry and Therapy. *Semin Neurol.* 2025 May;45(3):368-382.
[24] Winkelman JW, Berkowski JA, DelRosso LM, et al. Treatment of restless legs syndrome and periodic limb movement disorder: an American Academy of Sleep Medicine clinical practice guideline. *J Clin Sleep Med.* 2025 Jan 1;21(1):137–152.
[25] Allen RP, Picchietti DL, Auerbach M, et al. Evidence-based and consensus clinical practice guidelines for the iron treatment of restless legs syndrome/Willis-Ekbom disease in adults and children: an IRLSSG task force report. *Sleep Med.* 2018 Jan;41:27–44.
[26] Allen RP, Picchietti DL, Auerbach M, et al. Evidence-based and consensus clinical practice guidelines for the iron treatment of restless legs syndrome/Willis-Ekbom disease in adults and children: an IRLSSG task force report. *Sleep Med.* 2018 Jan;41:27–44.
[27] Zhang W, Zhao Y. Global Dietary Magnesium Deficiency: Prevalence, Underlying Causes, Health Consequences, and Strategic Solutions. *Int J Vit Nutr Res.* 2025 Dec;95(6):46828.
[28] DiNicolantonio JJ, O'Keefe JH, Wilson W. Subclinical magnesium deficiency: a principal driver of cardiovascular disease and a public health crisis. *Open Heart.* 2018 Jan;5(1):e000668.
[29] de Baaij JHF, Hoenderop JGJ, Bindels RJM. Magnesium in man: implications for health and disease. *Physiol Rev.* 2015 Jan;95(1):1–46.
[30] Wali SO, Abaalkhail BA, Alzahrani RA, et al. The association between vitamin D level and restless legs syndrome: a systematic review and meta-analysis. *Sleep Breath.* 2021 Jun;25(2):825–834.
[31] Hanna M, Jaqua E, Nguyen V, et al. B Vitamins: Functions and Uses in Medicine. *Perm J.* 2022 Jun 17;26(2):89–97.
[32] Patrick L.R. Restless legs syndrome: Pathophysiology and the role of iron and folate. *Altern Med Rev.* 2007;12:101–112.
[33] Xu XM, Ruan Jh, Tao T, et al. Role of vitamins in the pathogenesis and treatment of restless leg syndrome: A systematic review and meta-analysis. *PLOS One.* 2025;20(3):e0313571.
[34] Geng C, Yang Z, Xu P, et al. Possible association between vitamin B12 deficiency and restless legs syndrome. *Clin Neurol Neurosci.* 2022 Dec;223:107477.
[35] Collins JF, Prohaska JR, Knutson MD. Metabolic crossroads of iron and copper. *Nutr Rev.* 2010 Mar;68(3):133–147.
[36] Hurrell R, Egli I. Iron bioavailability and dietary reference values. *Am J Clin Nutr.* 2010 Dec;91(5):1461S–1467S.

[37] Fischer JA, Cherian AM, Bone JN, et al. The effects of oral ferrous bisglycinate supplementation on hemoglobin and ferritin concentrations in adults and children: a systematic review and meta-analysis of randomized controlled trials. *Nutr Rev*. 2023 Feb 2;81(8):904–920.
[38] Ruipubiological.com. The Bioavailability of Ferrous Bisglycinate: A Complete Overview. Accessed April 13, 2026 from: https://ruipubiological.com/07/06/post-83097/.
[39] Nemeth E, Ganz T. The role of hepcidin in iron metabolism. *Acta Haematol*. 2009;122(2-3):78–86.
[40] Kortman GAM, Raffatellu M, Swinkels DW, Tjalsma H. Nutritional iron turned inside out: intestinal stress from a gut microbial perspective. *FEMS Microbiol Rev*. 2014 Nov;38(6):1202–1234.
[41] Choi G, Bessman NJ. Iron at the crossroads of host–microbiome interactions in health and disease. *Nat Microbiol*. 2025 May 21;10(6):1282–1293.
[42] McEwen BS. Protective and damaging effects of stress mediators: central role of the brain. *Dialogues Clin Neurosci*. 2006 Jun;8(4):367–381.
[43] Irwin MR. Sleep and inflammation: partners in sickness and in health. *Nat Rev Immunol*. 2019 Nov;19(11):702–715.
[44] Lam JR, Schneider JL, Zhao W, Corley DA. Proton pump inhibitor and histamine-2 receptor antagonist use and iron deficiency. *Gastroenterology*. 2017 Mar;152(4):821–829.e1.
[45] Halfdanarson TR, Litzow MR, Murray JA. Hematologic manifestations of celiac disease. *Blood*. 2007 Jan 15;109(2):412–421.
[46] Stein J, Hartmann F, Dignass AU. Diagnosis and management of iron deficiency anemia in patients with inflammatory bowel disease. *Aliment Pharmacol Ther*. 2010 Jul;32(2):149–157.
[47] Muhsen K, Cohen D. Helicobacter pylori infection and iron stores: a systematic review and meta-analysis. *Helicobacter*. 2008 Oct;13(5):323–340.
[48] Aarts EO, van Wageningen B, Janssen IMC, Berends FJ. Prevalence of anemia and related deficiencies in the first year following laparoscopic gastric bypass for morbid obesity. *J Obes*. 2012;2012:193705.
[49] Lowe N, Gartner A, Dombrowski N, et al. Foot-strike Hemolysis: A Systematic Review of Long-Distance Runners. *Kans J Med*. 2024 Aug 27;17(Suppl 2):47.
[50] Winkelman JW, Armstrong MJ, Allen RP, et al. Practice guideline summary: treatment of restless legs syndrome in adults. *Neurology*. 2016 Dec 13;87(24):2585–2593.
[51] Allen RP, Picchietti DL, Garcia-Borreguero D, et al. Restless legs syndrome/Willis–Ekbom disease diagnostic criteria: updated International Restless Legs Syndrome Study Group (IRLSSG) consensus criteria—history, rationale, description, and significance. *Sleep Med*. 2014 Aug;15(8):860–873.
[52] Garcia-Borreguero D, Silber MH, Winkelman JW, et al. Guidelines for the first-line treatment of restless legs syndrome/Willis–Ekbom disease: an IRLSSG task force report. *Sleep Med*. 2016 Jan;21:1–11.
[53] Kang SG, Lee HJ, Jung SW, et al. Restless legs syndrome and antipsychotic use: a systematic review and meta-analysis. *J Clin Psychopharmacol*. 2019 Jun;39(3):273–281.
[54] Lam JR, Schneider JL, Zhao W, Corley DA. Proton pump inhibitor and histamine-2 receptor antagonist use and iron deficiency. *Gastroenterology*. 2017 Mar;152(4):821–829.e1.
[55] Auerbach M, Adamson JW. How we diagnose and treat iron deficiency anemia. *Am J Hematol*. 2016 Jan;91(1):31–38.

[56] Hurrell R, Egli I. Iron bioavailability and dietary reference values. *Am J Clin Nutr.* 2010 Dec;91(5):1461S–1467S.
[57] Hurrell R, Egli I. Iron bioavailability and dietary reference values. *Am J Clin Nutr.* 2010 Dec;91(5):1461S–1467S.
[58] Piskin E, Cianciosi D, Gulec S, et al. Iron Absorption: Factors, Limitations, and Improvement Methods. *ACS Omega.* 2022 Jun 10;7(24):20441–20456.
[59] Micha R, Wallace SK, Mozaffarian D. Red and processed meat consumption and risk of incident coronary heart disease, stroke, and diabetes mellitus: a systematic review and meta-analysis. *Circulation.* 2010 Mar 23;121(21):2271–2283.
[60] Li N, Zhao G, Wu W, et al. The Efficacy and Safety of Vitamin C for Iron Supplementation in Adult Patients With Iron Deficiency Anemia. *JAMA Netw Open.* 2020 Nov 2;3(11):e2023644.
[61] Ma Q, Kim EY, Kindsay EA, et al. Bioactive Dietary Polyphenols Inhibit Heme Iron Absorption in A Dose-Dependent Manner in Human Intestinal Caco-2 cells. *J Food Sci.* 2011 May 4;76(5):H143–H150.
[62] Hallberg L, Brune M, Rossander L. The role of vitamin C in iron absorption. *Int J Vitam Nutr Res Suppl.* 1989;30:103–108.
[63] Hurrell RF, Reddy MB, Cook JD. Inhibition of non-haem iron absorption in man by polyphenolic-containing beverages. *Br J Nutr.* 1999 Apr;81(4):289–295.
[64] Pineda O, Ashmead HD. Effectiveness of treatment of iron-deficiency anemia in infants and young children with ferrous bis-glycinate chelate. *J Appl Nutr.* 2001;53(1):1–13.
[65] Moretti D, Goede JS, Zeder C, et al. Oral iron supplements increase hepcidin and decrease iron absorption from daily or twice-daily doses in iron-depleted young women. *Blood.* 2015 May 14;126(17):1981–1989.
[66] Dhanvijay AD, Patidar V, Singh J, et al. Efficacy of daily versus alternate day oral iron supplementation for management of anaemia among general population: a systematic review and meta-analysis. *BMC Pharmacol Toxicol.* 2025 Aug 21;26:152.
[67] Camaschella C. Iron-deficiency anemia. *N Engl J Med.* 2015 May 7;372(19):1832–1843.
[68] Trotti LM, Becker LA. Iron for the treatment of restless legs syndrome. *Cochrane Database Syst Rev.* 2019 Jan 23;1(1):CD007834.
[69] Garcia-Borreguero D, Ferini-Strambi L, Kohnen R, et al. European guidelines on management of restless legs syndrome: report of a joint task force by the European Federation of Neurological Societies, the European Neurological Society, and the European Sleep Research Society. *Eur J Neurol.* 2012;19:1385-96.
[70] Winkelman JW, Armstrong MJ, Allen RP, Chaudhuri KR, Ondo W, Trenkwalder C, et al. Practice guideline summary: Treatment of restless legs syndrome in adults: Report of the Guideline Development, Dissemination, and Implementation Subcommittee of the American Academy of Neurology. *Neurology.* 2016;87(24):2585-93.
[71] Haskell MJ. The challenge to reach nutritional adequacy for vitamin A: beta-carotene bioavailability and conversion—evidence in humans. *Am J Clin Nutr.* 2012 May;96(5):1193S–1203S.
[72] Bochkov VN, Oskolkova OV, Birukov KG, et al. Generation and biological activities of oxidized phospholipids. *Antioxid Redox Signal.* 2010 Apr;12(8):1009–1059.
[73] Lucas L, Russell A, Keast R. Molecular mechanisms of inflammation. Anti-inflammatory benefits of virgin olive oil and the phenolic compound oleocanthal. *Curr Pharm Des.* 2011;17(8):754–768.

[74] Calder PC. Omega-3 fatty acids and inflammatory processes: from molecules to man. *Biochem Soc Trans.* 2017 Oct 15;45(5):1105–1115.
[75] Eyles DW, Smith S, Kinobe R, Hewison M, McGrath JJ. Distribution of the vitamin D receptor and 1α-hydroxylase in human brain. *J Chem Neuroanat.* 2005 Jan;29(1):21–30.
[76] Cui X, Gooch H, Groves NJ, Sah P, Burne THJ, Eyles DW, McGrath JJ. Vitamin D and the brain: key questions for future research. *J Steroid Biochem Mol Biol.* 2015 Jan;148:305–309.
[77] Santangelo C, Varì R, Scazzocchio B, et al. Polyphenols, intracellular signalling and inflammation. *Ann Ist Super Sanita.* 2007;43(4):394–405.
[78] Basu A, Rhone M, Lyons TJ. Berries: emerging impact on cardiovascular health. *Nutr Rev.* 2010 Mar;68(3):168–177.
[79] Katz DL, Doughty K, Ali A. Cocoa and chocolate in human health and disease. *Antioxid Redox Signal.* 2011 Sep 15;15(10):2779–2811.
[80] Aggarwal BB, Harikumar KB. Potential therapeutic effects of curcumin, the anti-inflammatory agent, against neurodegenerative, cardiovascular, pulmonary, metabolic, autoimmune and neoplastic diseases. *Int J Biochem Cell Biol.* 2009 Jan;41(1):40–59.
[81] Wastyk HC, Fragiadakis GK, Perelman D, et al. Gut-microbiota-targeted diets modulate human immune status. *Cell.* 2021 Jan 21;184(16):4137–4153.e14.
[82] Plaza-Díaz J, Ruiz-Ojeda FJ, Vilchez-Padial LM, Gil A. Evidence of the anti-inflammatory effects of probiotics and synbiotics in intestinal chronic diseases. *Nutrients.* 2017 Jun 30;9(6):555.
[83] Efthymakis K, Neri M. The role of Zinc L-Carnosine in the prevention and treatment of gastrointestinal mucosal disease in humans: a review. *Clin Res Hepatol Gastroenterol.* 2022 Aug-Sep;46(7):101954.
[84] Black PH. The inflammatory response is an integral part of the stress response: implications for atherosclerosis, insulin resistance, type II diabetes and metabolic syndrome X. *Brain Behav Immun.* 2003 Oct;17(5):350–364.
[85] Gleeson M, Bishop NC, Stensel DJ, Lindley MR, Mastana SS, Nimmo MA. The anti-inflammatory effects of exercise: mechanisms and implications for the prevention and treatment of disease. *Nat Rev Immunol.* 2011 Sep;11(9):607–615.
[86] Calderone A, Latella D, Impellizzeri F, et al. Neurobiological Changes Induced by Mindfulness and Meditation: A Systematic Review. *Biomedicines.* 2024 Nov 15;12(11):2613.
[87] Samoraj A, Zajaczkowski J, Krzeszowska P, et al. Therapeutic Effects of Forest Bathing on Human Health: A Systematic Review. *J Education Health Sport.* 2025 Jun;82:60242.
[88] Yang YC, Schorpp K, Harris KM. Social support, social strain and inflammation: Evidence from a national longitudinal study of U.S. adults. *Soc Sci Med.* 2014 Feb 14;107:124–135.
[89] Engert LC, Besedovsky L. Sleep and inflammation: a bidirectional relationship. *Springer Nature Link.* 2025 Jan;29:3-9.
[90] Huang X, Sun X, Wang Q, et al. Structural insights into the diverse actions of magnesium on NMDA receptors. *Neron.* 2025 Apr 2;113(7):P1006-18.
[91] Maier JAM, Locatelli L, Fedele G, et al. Magnesium and the Brain: A Focus on Neuroinflammation and Neurodegeneration. *Int J Mol Sci.* 2022 Dec 23;24(1):223.
[92] Al Alawi AM, Majoni SW, Falkammar H, et al. Magnesium and Human Health: Perspectives and Research Directions. *Int J Endocrinol.* 2018 Apr 16;2018:9041694.
[93] Rosanoff A, Weaver CM, Rude RK. Suboptimal magnesium status in the United States: are the health consequences underestimated? *Nutr Rev.* 2012 Mar;70(3):153–164.

[94] Zhang W, Zhao Y. Global Dietary Magnesium Deficiency: Prevalence, Underlying Causes, Health Consequences, and Strategic Solutions. *Int J Vitam Nutr Res.* 2025 Dec 25;95(6):46828.
[95] Zhang W, Zhao Y. Global Dietary Magnesium Deficiency: Prevalence, Underlying Causes, Health Consequences, and Strategic Solutions. *Int J Vitamin Nutr Res.* 2025 Dec;95(6):46828.
[96] Drummartin Clinic. Magnesium: A much-overlooked mineral. Accessed April 15, 2026 from: https://drummartinclinic.ie/magnesium-deficiency/.
[97] Lopresti AL, Smith SJ. The effects of magnesium L-threonate (Magtein®) on cognitive performance and sleep quality in adults: a randomised, double-blind, placebo-controlled trial. *Front Nutr.* 2026 Jan 12;12:1729164.
[98] Firoz M, Graber M. Bioavailability of US commercial magnesium preparations. *Magnes Res.* 2001 Dec;14(4):257-62.
[99] Bannai M, Kawai N. The effects of glycine on subjective daytime performance in partially sleep-restricted healthy volunteers. *Front Neurol.* 2012 Oct 23;3:61.
[100] Kawai N, Sakai N, Okuro M, et al. The Sleep-Promoting and Hypothermic Effects of Glycine are Mediated by NMDA Receptors in the Suprachiasmatic Nucleus. *Neuropsychopharmacology*. 2015 Jan 14;40(6):1405–1416.
[101] Ochoa-de la Paz L, Zenteno E, Gulias-Canizo R, et al. Taurine and GABA neurotransmitter receptors, a relationship with therapeutic potential? *Expert Rev Neurother.* 2019 Jan:289-91.
[102] Ramirez-Guerro S, Guardo-Maya S, Medina-Rincon GJ, et al. Taurine and Astrocytes: A Homeostatic and Neuroprotective Relationship. *Front Mol Neurosci.* 2022 Jul 5:15:937789.
[103] Manyam BV. Mucuna pruriens in Parkinson's disease: a double blind clinical and pharmacological study. *J Neurol Neurosurg Psychiatry*. 2004 Dec;75(12):1672–1677.
[104] Hammound F, Ismail A, Zaher R, et al. Mucuna pruriens Treatment for Parkinson Disease: A Systematic Review of Clinical Trials. *Parkinsons Dis.* 2025 Aug 18;2025:1319419.
[105] Sohutskay DO, Suen RM, Ali F, et al. Dopamine Dysregulation Syndrome Presenting as Overuse of Mucuna pruriens Levodopa Supplement. *J Mov Disord.* 2024 May 21;17(3):357–359.
[106] Silvani MI, Werder R, Perret C. The influence of blue light on sleep, performance and wellbeing in young adults: A systematic review. *Front Physiol.* 2022 Aug 16;13:943108.
[107] Hartley N, MCLachlan CS. Aromas Influencing the GABAergic System. *Molecules.* 2022;27(8):2414.
[108] Milanos S, Elsharif S, Janzen D, et al. Metabolic Products of Linalool and Modulation of GABAA Receptors. *Front Chem.* 2017 Jun 21;5:46.
[109] Hashimoto M, Takahashi K, Ohta T. Inhibitory effects of linalool, an essential oil component of lavender, on nociceptive TRPA1 and voltage-gated Ca2+ channels in mouse sensory neurons. *Biochem Biophys Rep.* 2023 Apr 12;34:101468.
[110] El Alaoui C, Chemin J, Fechtali T, et al. Modulation of T-type Ca2+ channels by Lavender and Rosemary extracts. *PLOS One.* 2017 Oct 26;12(10):e0186864.
[111] Linck VM, da Silva AL, Figueiró M, et al. Inhaled linalool-induced sedation in mice. *Phytomedicine.* 2009 Mar;16(4):303–307.
[112] Aprotosoaie AC, Hancianu M, Costache II, et al. Linalool: a review on a key odorant molecule with valuable biological properties. *Flavour Fragr J.* 2014 Mar 11;29(4):193-219.
[113] Satou T, Koutoku Y, Odata K. Effect of Lavender Essential Oil Topical Treatment on the Autonomic Nervous System in Human Subjects Without Olfactory Influence: A Pilot Study. *Nat Prod Commun.* 2024 Aug;19(8).

[114] Jäger W, Buchbauer G, Jirovetz L, et al. Percutaneous absorption of lavender oil from a massage oil. *J Soc Cosmetic Chemists*. 1992;43:49-54.
[115] Yap WS, Dolzhenko AV, Jalal Z, et al. Efficacy and safety of lavender essential oil (Silexan) capsules among patients suffering from anxiety disorders: A network meta-analysis. *Sci Rep*. 2019 Dec 2;9:18042.
[116] Dold M, Bartova L, Volz HP, et al. Efficacy of Silexan in patients with anxiety disorders: a meta-analysis of randomized, placebo-controlled trials. *Nature Link*. 2023 Jan 30;273:1615-28.
[117] Schuwald AM, Noldner M, Wilmes T, et al. Lavender Oil-Potent Anxiolytic Properties via Modulating Voltage Dependent Calcium Channels. *PLoS One*. 2013 Apr 29;8(4):e59998.
[118] Baldinger P, Hoflich AS, Mitterhauser M, et al. Effects of Silexan on the Serotonin-1A Receptor and Microstructure of the Human Brain: A Randomized, Placebo-Controlled, Double-Blind, Cross-Over Study with Molecular and Structural Neuroimaging. *Int J Neurophsychopharmacol*. 2015 Feb;18(4).
[119] Darwin Nutrition. Roman chamomile: benefits, dosage, contraindications. Accessed April 18, 2026 from: https://www.darwin-nutrition.fr/en/active/roman-chamomile/.
[120] Landema. Isobutyl angelate. Accessed April 18, 2026 from: https://landema.com/en-us/lexicon/molecular-guide/isobutyl-angelate.
[121] Sandor Z, Mottaghipisheh J, Veres K, et al. Evidence Supports Tradition: The in Vitro Effects of Roman Chamomile on Smooth Muscles. *Front Pharmacol*. 2018 Apr 6;9:323.
[122] Johnson SA. *Medicinal Essential Oils: The Science and Practice of Evidence-based Essential Oil Therapy*, second edition. 2023.
[123] Prerna, Chadha J, Khullar L, et al. A comprehensive review on the pharmacological prospects of Terpinen-4-ol: From nature to medicine and beyond. *Fitoterapia*. 2024 Jul;176:106051.
[124] Singh S, Mishra A. Linalool: Therapeutic Indication And Their Multifaceted Biomedical Applications.
Drug Res (Stuttg). 2024 Jul;74(6):255-268.
[125] Johnson SA. *Co2 Aromatics, Medicinal Herbs, and Targeted Nutraceutical for Healing and Greater Wellness*. 2023.
[126] Moussaieff A, Rimmerman N, Bregman T, et al. Incensole acetate, an incense component, elicits psychoactivity by activating TRPV3 channels in the brain. *FASEB J*. 2008 Aug;22(8):3024–3034.
[127] von Schoen-Angerer T, Deckers B, Henes J, et al. Effect of topical rosemary essential oil on Raynaud phenomenon in systemic sclerosis. *Complement Ther Med*. 2018 Oct;40:191-94.
[128] Johnson SA, Rodriguez D, Allred K, et al. A Systematic Review of Essential Oils and the Endocannabinoid System: A Connection Worthy of Further Exploration. *Evidence-Based Complement Altern Med*. 2020 Mat 16;(25):1-13.
[129] Zhang N, Chen J, Dong W, et al. The Effect of Copaiba Oil Odor on Anxiety Relief in Adults under Mental Workload: A Randomized Controlled Trial. *Evidence-Based Complement Altern Med*. 2022 Mar 20;2022:3874745.
[130] Cinar V, Bag MF, Aslan M, et al. Impact of different exercise modalities on neuroendocrine well-being markers among university students: a study of renalase and catecholamine responses. *Front Physiol*. 2025 Apr 30;16:2025.
[131] Cerqueira E, Marinho DA, Neiva HP, et al. Inflammatory Effects of High and Moderate Intensity Exercise—A Systematic Review. *Front Physiol*. 2020 Jan 8;10:2019.

[132] Zapalac K, Miller M, Champagne FA, et al. The effects of physical activity on sleep architecture and mood in naturalistic environments. *Sci Rep.* 2024 Mar 7;14:5637.
[133] He S, Hasler BP, Chakravorty S. Alcohol and sleep-related problems. *Curr Opin Psychol.* 2019 Aug;30:117–122.
[134] Rivilin RS. Magnesium deficiency and alcohol intake: mechanisms, clinical significance and possible relation to cancer development (a review). *J Am Coll Nutr.* 1994 Oct;13(5):416-23.
[135] Pu S, Zhuang Z, Liu N, et al. Research progress on the relationship between Helicobacter pylori infection and iron deficiency anemia. *Front Microbiol.* 2025 Mar 25;16:1552630.
[136] Li Y, MMed, Choi H, et al. Global prevalence of Helicobacter pylori infection between 1980 and 2022: a systematic review and meta-analysis. *The Lancet Gastroenterol Hepatol.* 2023 Jun;8(6):553-64.
[137] Carboni L. Active Folate Versus Folic Acid: The Role of 5-MTHF (Methylfolate) in Human Health. *Integr Med (Encinitas).* 2022 Jul;21(3):36–41.
[138] Moll S, Varga EA. Homocysteine and MTHFR Mutations. *Circulation.* 2015 Jul 7;132(1).
[139] Grody WW, Griffin JH, Taylor AK, et al. American College of Medical Genetics consensus statement on factor V Leiden mutation testing. *Genet Med.* 2001 Mar-Apr;3(2):139-48.
[140] Antoniades C, Antonopoulos AS, Tousoulis D, et al. Homocysteine and coronary atherosclerosis: from folate fortification to the recent clinical trials. *Eur Heart J.* 2009 Jan;30(1):6-15.
[141] Lynch B. The Folic Acid Brain Problem No One Explains. Accessed April 19, 20206 from: https://www.youtube.com/watch?v=o9xfbdrna9g.
[142] Mazokopakis EE, Papadomanolaki MG, Papadakis JA. The effects of folinic acid and l-methylfolate supplementation on serum total homocysteine levels in healthy adults. *Clin Nutr ESPEN.* 2023 Dec;58:14-20.
[143] Yang Q, Li L, Chen Q, et al. Association studies of variants in MEIS1, BTBD9 and MAP2K5/SKOR1 with restless legs syndrome in a U.S. population. *Sleep Med.* 2011 Sep;12(8):800–804.

Index

F

G

H

I

K

L

M

N

O

P

Q

R

S

T

U

V

W

Z